Nephrology

Nursing Care

THE COMPLETE GUIDE

ALEXANDRE CAREWELL

Table of Contents

« Nephrology doesn't just study the kidneys, it probes the very heart of our internal balance, ensuring that every drop translates into renewed health. »

INTRODUCTION

The importance of nephrology in the medical landscape.

Nephrology, although sometimes tucked away in the shadows of more 'high-profile' medical specialities, occupies a crucial place in the global panorama of medicine. This discipline, which focuses on the study, diagnosis and treatment of kidney disease, is the silent guardian of our bodies' internal balance. Every function of our kidneys is a testament to natural ingenuity, filtering waste, balancing fluid levels and regulating electrolytes. If this biochemical symphony were to be interrupted, the consequences for the individual would be catastrophic.

Nephrology stands out in the medical landscape not only for its technical complexity, but also for its closeness to the patient. Chronic kidney disease, for example, requires regular care and monitoring, forging a close bond between the patient, the nephrologist and the nursing team. These repeated interactions offer a unique perspective on the prolonged nature of medical care and the importance of a relationship based on trust.

Moreover, the importance of nephrology extends beyond its disciplinary boundaries. It plays a central role in the management of many common pathologies, including diabetes and hypertension, two of the main culprits in kidney failure. In other words, the work of nephrologists and nephrology nurses does not simply stop at kidney function, but forms part of a broader framework of prevention, care and treatment in general medicine.

In addition, technological advances, particularly in the field of dialysis, reflect the dynamic role played by nephrology in the adoption and adaptation of medical technology. Continuous innovation in renal care demonstrates the extent to which this speciality is at the cutting edge of modern medicine.

So, although it may seem specialised and sometimes isolated, nephrology is in fact a fundamental pillar of medicine. It is a reminder of the interconnectedness of our body systems, the vitality of prevention, and the marvel of medical technology. In the grand scheme of medicine, nephrology is an essential speciality, a constant reminder of how precious every organ, every cell and every moment is in the delicate dance of life.

The pivotal role of the nephrology nurse.

The nephrology nurse is at the heart of a medical universe where the technical nature of care blends with the depth of human relationships. Playing a pivotal role, this key player is often the first line of contact for patients with kidney disease, serving not only as a carer, but also as a guide, educator and sometimes even confidant.

Nephrology care, particularly dialysis, requires technical expertise and specific skills. Nurses must ensure that machines are working properly, that medication dosages are correct, and that all procedures are followed to the letter. A minor error can have major consequences, making vigilance and precision essential in this role.

However, beyond this technical expertise, it is in the human accompaniment that the nephrology nurse truly shines. Patients with chronic renal failure or other kidney conditions are often faced with long-term treatments, lifestyle changes and a multitude of emotions, ranging from fear to frustration. This is where the nurse comes in, offering emotional support, answering questions, allaying fears and helping to manage expectations.

Education also plays a predominant role in this speciality. Nurses inform patients about their treatments, guide them in managing their diet, make them aware of the importance of taking their medication regularly and prepare them for possible kidney transplants. This educational aspect is a key element in helping patients to take control of their own health and improve their quality of life.

Finally, the nephrology nurse is often the link between the patient and the nephrologist. They pass on essential information, coordinate care and ensure that the care pathway is smooth and efficient. They also work closely with other specialists, such as dieticians and social workers, to ensure that patients receive comprehensive care.

In the vast world of nephrology, the nurse is a compass, an anchor and a guardian. While technically qualified, their role extends far beyond the purely clinical to embrace a profoundly human dimension, making them an invaluable ally for every patient navigating the often tumultuous waters of kidney disease.

Chapter 1:
NEPHROLOGY - AN INTRODUCTION

Understanding kidneys: anatomy and physiology.

The kidneys, those two bean-shaped organs on either side of the spine, are essential to life. Although they are perhaps not as frequently mentioned as the heart or lungs in current discussions on health, their role in maintaining the body's internal balance is just as crucial. To understand their importance, we need to delve into the anatomy and physiology of these remarkable structures.

Kidney anatomy
Location: The kidneys are located in the lumbar region, just below the rib cage, on either side of the spinal column. They are protected by the rib cage and a layer of fat.
External structure: Each kidney is approximately 10 to 12 cm long, 5 to 7 cm wide and 2 to 3 cm thick. The concave part of the kidney, called the hilum, is where the ureter, blood vessels and nerves enter and exit the organ.
Internal structure: Internally, the kidney is divided into several regions:
- The **cortex**: the outer layer containing numerous nephrons, the functional units of the kidneys.
- The **medulla**, divided into renal pyramids, which contains collecting tubes leading to structures called calyces, which collect the urine produced by the nephrons.

Kidney physiology

The kidneys perform many essential functions:

- **Blood filtration**: Every day, the kidneys filter around 180 litres of blood, eliminating waste and excess fluids to produce around 1 to 2 litres of urine.
- **Electrolyte regulation**: The kidneys regulate the concentrations of sodium, potassium, calcium and other ions in the blood, ensuring the stability of the body's internal environment.
- **Regulation of blood pressure**: By secreting the hormone renin, the kidneys play an essential role in regulating blood pressure.
- **Production of erythropoietin**: This hormone stimulates the production of red blood cells in the bone marrow when oxygen levels in the blood are low.
- **Metabolism of vitamin D**: The kidneys convert vitamin D into its active form, which is essential for the absorption of calcium by the intestines.
- **Acid-base balance**: The kidneys regulate blood pH by excreting hydrogen ions and reabsorbing bicarbonate.

Through these functions, the kidneys play an active role in maintaining a stable internal environment, known as homeostasis. This balance is essential for cells and organs to function properly. Without healthy kidneys, this balance would be disturbed, threatening the optimal functioning of the body as a whole. So to understand the kidneys is to recognise the complexity and beauty of physiological design, and to appreciate their silent but vital role in our daily well-being.

Common pathologies in nephrology.

Nephrology is a medical speciality dedicated to the study, diagnosis and treatment of kidney disease. The kidneys, as the organs responsible for filtering blood and regulating many of the body's essential functions, can be affected by a multitude of pathologies. Some of these are common and deserve special attention because of their prevalence and potential impact on health.

1. Renal failure
   • **Acute renal failure (ARF): This is a** sudden and rapid loss of kidney function, often due to kidney damage, severe dehydration, certain drugs or sepsis.
   • **Chronic kidney disease (CKD)**: This condition is characterised by a gradual and irreversible loss of kidney function. Common causes include diabetes, high blood pressure and chronic glomerulonephritis.

2. Glomerulonephritis
This is an inflammation of the glomeruli, the small filtration units in the kidneys. It can be acute or chronic and can result from infections, autoimmune diseases or other causes.

3. Diabetic nephropathy
This is a common complication of diabetes and is one of the main causes of chronic kidney failure. It is due to damage to the blood vessels in the kidneys caused by high blood sugar levels.

4. Renal lithiasis (kidney stones)
These are solid masses of crystals that develop inside the kidneys. These stones can cause pain and obstruct the flow of urine.

5. Polycystic kidney disease
This is a genetic condition in which numerous cysts, or fluid-filled sacs, develop in the kidneys, compromising their function.

6. Nephrotic syndrome
This is a set of symptoms that includes high proteinuria (excessive protein in the urine), hypoalbuminemia (low albumin concentration in the blood) and oedema.

7. Renovascular hypertension
This is a form of high blood pressure caused by narrowing of the renal arteries.

8. Pyelonephritis
This is a kidney infection often caused by bacteria that spread from the bladder to the kidneys.

9. Hereditary diseases
In addition to polycystic kidney disease, there are other genetic conditions, such as Alport syndrome, which affect kidney function.

10. Renal toxicity
Many drugs and toxins can damage the kidneys if taken in large quantities or over a prolonged period.

The management of these diseases often requires a multidisciplinary approach involving nephrologists, specialist nurses, dieticians and other healthcare professionals. Prevention, early detection and appropriate treatment are essential to minimise complications and improve the quality of life of patients with kidney disease.

The journey of a nephrology patient.

A nephrology patient's journey is a complex medical trajectory, shaped by the nature of their kidney disease, their symptoms, the interventions required and their general state of health. This journey, often punctuated by moments of uncertainty, adaptation and resilience, highlights the importance of comprehensive, coordinated, patient-centred care.

1. Symptoms and initial consultation
The process often begins with the appearance of unexplained symptoms such as fatigue, oedema, frothy urine or back pain. Patients can then consult their GP, who will prescribe further tests if these signs appear.

2. Initial examination and diagnosis
Blood tests, urine analysis and a kidney ultrasound scan may be carried out. If an abnormality is detected, the GP will refer the patient to a nephrologist for a more detailed examination. The precise diagnosis of kidney disease is established thanks to these investigations and sometimes a kidney biopsy.

3. Education and initial care
Once the diagnosis has been made, a phase of education begins. The nephrologist, supported by a team of specialist nurses, informs the patient about the disease, possible treatments and recommended lifestyle changes. This stage is crucial if patients are to understand their condition and adhere to the treatment.

4. Specific treatment
Depending on the nature and severity of the disease, treatment may vary:
  • Specific medication to control the progression of the disease.

- Dietary changes to protect renal function.
- Dialysis, if renal function is severely impaired.
- Renal transplantation for advanced renal failure.

5. Regular monitoring
Nephrology patients require regular follow-up to assess the progress of their disease, adjust treatments and manage any complications. These regular appointments are essential for monitoring the patient's state of health.

6. Multidisciplinary support
In addition to nephrologists, other professionals are involved in the patient's care: dieticians to adjust the diet, psychologists for emotional support, social workers for administrative assistance, and physiotherapists to manage mobility.

7. Transition to other care
Depending on how the disease progresses, a patient may require more intensive care, such as a switch to more frequent dialysis or a kidney transplant. These transitions are closely managed to ensure continuity of care.

8. Continuing education and rehabilitation
Over time, the patient's needs may change. The education sessions are renewed and adapted to accompany them through each phase of their illness.
A nephrology patient's journey is a medical and human one. At every stage, close collaboration between the patient, his or her family and the medical team is essential to ensure the best possible outcome and improve quality of life.

Chapter 2:
ROLE AND RESPONSIBILITIES
OF THE NEPHROLOGY NURSE

The day-to-day life of a nurse
in nephrology.

Nephrology nurses play a central role in the care of patients suffering from kidney disease. Their role goes far beyond the simple administration of care; they are a real pillar of patient support, acting as educators, supporters and coordinators. The daily life of these professionals is punctuated by a multitude of tasks, making it as demanding as it is rewarding.

1. Treatment administration
Nurses are often on the front line when it comes to administering medicines, whether orally, intravenously or otherwise. In nephrology, this may also include managing dialysis treatments.

2. Monitoring dialysis
For dialysis patients, the nurse prepares and monitors the machine, connects the patient, monitors the patient's condition during treatment and manages any potential problems. Dialysis is a demanding treatment that requires constant attention.

3. Medical follow-up
Nurses regularly measure patients' vital signs, assess their well-being, monitor potential side effects of treatment and report any abnormalities to the nephrologist.

4. Patient education

Nurses play a crucial role in patient education. They inform them about their disease, treatments, recommended lifestyle changes and self-monitoring techniques.

5. Emotional support

Faced with a chronic illness, many patients may feel anxious, depressed or discouraged. Nurses are often the first point of contact and support for these patients, offering a listening ear and advice.

6. Coordination with the medical team

Nurses work in close collaboration with nephrologists, dieticians, social workers and other members of the medical team to ensure comprehensive, coordinated patient care.

7. Technical procedures

This may include inserting catheters, taking blood samples, managing vascular access for dialysis or post-transplant monitoring for patients who have received a new kidney.

8. Administrative tasks

Like all healthcare professionals, nephrology nurses must also manage administrative tasks, such as updating medical records, ordering medicines and coordinating appointments.

9. Further training

Medicine is constantly evolving. Nurses therefore need regular training to keep up to date with the latest techniques, treatments and recommendations in the field of nephrology.

The role of the nephrology nurse is multifaceted. It requires both advanced technical skills and a great capacity for empathy. These professionals are often at the heart of the patient's medical experience, accompanying them at every stage of their nephrology journey, making them essential players in the care of these patients.

Interprofessional collaboration: working with a multidisciplinary team.

Patient care in nephrology, as in many other medical fields, does not rely solely on the expertise of a single healthcare professional. It requires close collaboration between different specialists, each of whom brings his or her own specific knowledge and know-how to the task of providing patients with the best possible overall care. Interprofessional collaboration is at the heart of this approach, ensuring that every aspect of the patient's health is taken into account.

1. The pivotal role of the nephrologist
The nephrologist is a specialist in kidney disease. They diagnose the disease, advise on the best treatment and monitor its progress. He or she usually coordinates the multidisciplinary team.

2. The nephrology nurse
In addition to direct care, nurses play a central role in patient education, daily monitoring, care coordination and emotional support.

3. The dietician
Kidney disease often has specific dietary implications. The dietician advises patients on their diet, depending on the progression of their disease and the treatments prescribed.

4. The social worker
It supports patients and their families in dealing with the non-medical challenges associated with the disease, such

as financial problems, access to care or employment concerns.

5. The pharmacist
As experts in medicines, pharmacists advise on dosage, drug interactions and side effects. They work closely with the nephrologist to ensure that the patient receives the most appropriate treatment.

6. The psychologist
Faced with a chronic illness, many patients experience anxiety, depression or stress. The psychologist helps them to manage these emotions and suggests coping strategies.

7. The physiotherapist
For patients with mobility difficulties or pain, the physiotherapist offers exercises and techniques to improve their quality of life.

8. The vascular surgeon
For patients requiring dialysis, it is often necessary to create a vascular access. The vascular surgeon works in collaboration with the nephrologist.

9. Communication and coordination
The key to successful interprofessional collaboration lies in fluid and regular communication between team members. Regular multidisciplinary meetings, shared reporting and ongoing training are essential to ensure smooth and effective care.

Interprofessional collaboration ensures that patients benefit from a holistic approach, where every aspect of their health is taken into account. In an increasingly specialised medical world, this multidisciplinary approach is crucial to providing patients with comprehensive care, focused on their needs and well-being.

Administrative responsibilities and documentation.

In the world of healthcare, and particularly in nephrology, documentation and administrative responsibilities play a crucial role. Not only do they guarantee optimal patient care, they also ensure that care is traceable and that legal and ethical obligations are met. Nephrology nurses, like all healthcare professionals, have to juggle their direct care duties with these administrative responsibilities.

1. Keeping medical records
The medical file is the patient's central monitoring tool. It contains the history of consultations, test results, medical prescriptions and any other information relevant to the patient's health. Nurses must ensure that this file is constantly updated, including their observations and interventions.

2. Ordering and managing medicines and equipment
Nephrology care often requires the use of specific drugs and equipment, such as dialysis equipment. Nurses must ensure that these are available, manage stocks and sometimes order new equipment or medicines.

3. Appointment coordination
The nurse often plays a role in coordinating medical appointments, whether for regular consultations, dialysis sessions or other specialist examinations.

4. Relationships and communication with other healthcare professionals
Nurses are often required to communicate with other members of the medical team, whether through written reports, oral accounts or coordination meetings. These exchanges ensure that patients receive harmonious, coordinated care.

5. Compliance with standards and regulations

Healthcare is governed by a whole range of standards and regulations, covering hygiene, safety, confidentiality and ethics. Nurses must have a thorough knowledge of these and ensure that they are scrupulously respected.

6. Training and continuing education

The healthcare field is constantly evolving. This means that nurses need to keep up to date with new techniques, the latest drugs and innovative care methods. This ongoing training must also be documented.

7. Participation in clinical research

In some establishments, nurses may be involved in clinical research projects. This involves precise documentation, following protocols and communicating with research teams.

8. Assessing the quality of care

To guarantee optimal care, many establishments are introducing regular assessments of the quality of care. Nurses often take part in these assessments, both as assessors and as those being assessed.

At first glance, administrative and documentation responsibilities may seem far removed from the core of a nurse's job. However, they are essential for guaranteeing the safety, efficiency and quality of the care provided to patients. In an increasingly complex medical world, mastering them is an essential skill for all healthcare professionals.

Chapter 3:
TECHNIQUES
AND STANDARD PROCEDURES

Dialysis: principles and types

Dialysis is an essential medical technique in the field of nephrology, used to purify the blood of patients whose kidneys are not functioning or are functioning insufficiently. It removes waste products, excess fluid and electrolytes from the blood, performing a function normally carried out by healthy kidneys. Let's delve into the principles and types of dialysis to gain a better understanding of this vital procedure.

1. Principles of dialysis
The kidneys act as filters for our body, eliminating waste and excess water to form urine. When the kidneys lose this filtering capacity, the blood becomes loaded with toxic waste and excess fluid. Dialysis is used to replace this failing kidney function. It is based on the principle of diffusion, where molecules move from an area of high concentration to an area of low concentration, and osmosis, for the transfer of water.

2. Haemodialysis
- **Principle**: Haemodialysis is the most common type of dialysis. The patient's blood is pumped out of the body to a dialysis machine, which filters it before returning it to the body.
- **Vascular access**: To allow blood to circulate, a vascular access is created, often in the arm. This may be a fistula, a graft or a catheter.

- **Frequency**: Haemodialysis is generally carried out three times a week, with each session lasting approximately 3 to 5 hours.

3. Peritoneal dialysis
- **Principle**: In peritoneal dialysis, the blood is cleaned inside the body. The peritoneal membrane, which lines the abdomen, is used as a natural filter. A dialysis solution is introduced into the abdomen through a catheter and, after a certain period of time, it is evacuated, taking with it waste products and excess fluid.
- Types :
    - **Continuous ambulatory peritoneal dialysis (CAPD)**: Fluid exchanges are carried out manually, generally 4 times a day.
    - **Automated peritoneal dialysis (APD)**: A machine carries out fluid exchanges during the night while the patient sleeps.

4. Advantages and disadvantages
Each type of dialysis has its advantages and disadvantages. Haemodialysis requires frequent visits to a dialysis centre and can be more restrictive for the patient. Peritoneal dialysis, on the other hand, offers greater freedom, as it can be carried out at home, but requires rigorous asepsis and the ability to manage exchanges yourself.

5. Choice of method
The choice of dialysis method depends on a number of factors: the patient's overall health, remaining kidney function, lifestyle, ability to manage treatment at home and personal preferences. An in-depth discussion with the nephrologist is essential to choosing the best option.

Dialysis is a life-saving process for many patients suffering from chronic renal failure. Although it does not replace all kidney functions, it allows patients to continue to live a productive life while managing their kidney disease.

Haemodialysis

Haemodialysis is one of the most common methods of dialysis used to treat chronic renal failure. It allows the blood to be filtered to eliminate waste products, toxins and excess fluid, thus partially reproducing the function of the kidneys. Treatment is essential for people whose kidneys are no longer able to perform this vital task. Let's take a look at the detailed aspects of haemodialysis.

1. How haemodialysis works
During a haemodialysis session, the patient's blood is pumped out of the body into a haemodialysis machine. This machine includes a dialyser, or "artificial kidney", which filters the blood. Once cleaned, the blood is returned to the patient's body.

2. Vascular access
A key aspect of haemodialysis is the establishment of a strong and durable vascular access to allow efficient blood flow between the patient and the machine. Types of access include:
- **Arteriovenous fistula (AVF): This is a** surgical connection between an artery and a vein, usually in the arm. It is preferred for its durability and lower risk of infection.
- **Graft**: A synthetic tube is used to connect an artery to a vein.
- **Catheter**: When haemodialysis is required on a short-term basis, a catheter can be inserted into a large vein in the neck or chest.

3. Frequency and duration

A typical haemodialysis session lasts around 3 to 5 hours and is generally required three times a week. However, the duration and frequency may vary according to the patient's needs.

4. Dialysis environment

Haemodialysis is most often carried out in a specialist dialysis centre. Some centres offer nocturnal haemodialysis, allowing patients to dialyse while they sleep. It is also possible to carry out haemodialysis at home, after appropriate training.

5. Advantages and disadvantages

- Advantages :
- Scheduled treatments to allow other activities to be planned.
- Close medical supervision during treatment.
- Release of days without pay.
- Disadvantages :
- Frequent visits to the dialysis centre.
- Possible post-dialysis fatigue.
- Food and water restrictions.

6. Potential complications

As with any medical procedure, haemodialysis carries risks. These include
- Muscle cramps
- Hypotension (low blood pressure)
- Infections
- Anemia
- Vascular access problems

7. Quality of life with haemodialysis

Living with haemodialysis requires lifestyle adjustments. Patients must manage their diet and water intake, take several medications and adhere to a strict dialysis schedule. However, with the right support and management, many patients lead active and fulfilling lives. Haemodialysis remains a mainstay of treatment for chronic renal failure. It offers a lifeline to millions of people around the world, enabling them to live despite advanced kidney disease.

Peritoneal dialysis

Peritoneal dialysis is an alternative to haemodialysis for the treatment of chronic renal failure. It uses the patient's peritoneal membrane, which lines the abdominal cavity, as a filter to eliminate waste, excess fluid and electrolytes. Usually performed at home, this technique offers patients greater autonomy. Let's take a closer look at the specific features of peritoneal dialysis.

1. Principle of peritoneal dialysis
Peritoneal dialysis involves the introduction of a special dialysis solution, generally rich in glucose, into the abdominal cavity. This solution draws waste products, electrolytes and excess fluid from the blood through the peritoneal membrane. After a certain period of time, known as the residence time, this 'used' solution is evacuated from the abdomen and replaced by a fresh solution.

2. Positioning the catheter
To allow the dialysis solution to enter and exit the body, a flexible catheter is surgically implanted in the abdominal wall. This procedure is generally straightforward and carried out on an outpatient basis or during a short stay in hospital.

3. Types of peritoneal dialysis
- Continuous ambulatory peritoneal dialysis (CAPD) :

- Performed manually by the patient or a carer.
- In general, it requires 4 exchanges a day, with the solution remaining in the abdomen for 4 to 6 hours before being exchanged.
- Automated peritoneal dialysis (APD) :
- Uses a machine, called a cycler, to carry out solution exchanges during the night while the patient is asleep.
- May need to be replaced manually during the day.

4. Advantages and disadvantages
- Advantages :
- Greater autonomy and flexibility.
- No repeated punctures as with haemodialysis.
- Better preservation of residual renal function.
- Fewer dietary restrictions.
- Disadvantages :
- Need to make daily exchanges.
- Risk of peritoneal infections.
- The sensation of having a "full" abdomen can be uncomfortable for some people.
- Possible weight gain due to glucose in the solution.

5. Monitoring and complications
Regular monitoring by a nephrologist and a healthcare team is essential. Patients must be alert to signs of infection and ensure that sterility is maintained when exchanges are carried out. Thorough initial training is essential to avoid complications, particularly peritoneal infection, which is the most common.

6. Transition and combination of treatments
Some patients start with peritoneal dialysis before moving on to haemodialysis, or vice versa, depending on the progression of their disease, their lifestyle or their

preferences. Others combine the two methods to best meet their needs.

Peritoneal dialysis is a valuable option for many patients suffering from kidney failure. It provides the necessary treatment while preserving a degree of independence and quality of life. With appropriate education and regular monitoring, it can be an effective and appropriate method of managing kidney failure.

Renal transplantation: before, during and after.

Kidney transplantation is considered to be the treatment of choice for many patients with end-stage renal disease. It offers a chance to lead a more normal life than dialysis. However, the procedure requires serious preparation, delicate surgery and rigorous post-operative monitoring. Let's explore the kidney transplant journey.

1. Before the transplant: preparation
   - **Assessment and eligibility**: Before being considered for transplantation, patients undergo a full medical assessment to determine their ability to tolerate the operation and the immunosuppressive drugs required afterwards.
   - **Finding a compatible donor**: This may be a living donor (usually a family member or friend) or a deceased donor. Blood and tissue tests are carried out to ensure compatibility.
   - **Psychological preparation**: Transplantation can have profound psychological effects. Psychological support is essential to help patients manage stress, fear and expectations.

2. During transplantation: the procedure
- **The operation**: The diseased kidney is not usually removed unless there are certain complications. The new kidney is placed in a different position, usually in the lower abdomen. The surgeon connects the artery and vein of the new kidney to the patient's blood vessels.
- **Launching the new kidney**: In many cases, the transplanted kidney begins to function immediately. However, sometimes it can take a few days or weeks before it is fully functional.

3. After the transplant: life with a new kidney
- **Immunosuppressive drugs**: To prevent rejection of the transplanted kidney, patients must take immunosuppressive drugs for the rest of their lives. These drugs reduce the activity of the immune system, making the patient more susceptible to infections.
- **Regular medical monitoring**: Frequent consultations with the nephrologist are necessary to monitor renal function, detect early signs of rejection and adjust medication.
- **Lifestyle**: Although quality of life generally improves after a transplant, it is essential to adopt a healthy lifestyle to protect the new kidney. This includes a balanced diet, regular exercise, avoiding alcohol and tobacco, and taking prescribed medication regularly.
- **Potential complications**: In addition to the risk of rejection, other complications may arise, including infections, cancers, cardiovascular disease and side-effects of medication.

Kidney transplantation is a journey with its challenges, hopes and rewards. Although it offers a new chance to lead a near-normal life, it requires constant responsibility and vigilance to preserve and protect the precious gift of a new kidney. With the right support and care, many kidney transplant patients lead long and fulfilling lives.

Catheter management and vascular access.

The management of catheters and vascular access is essential in nephrology, especially for those requiring regular dialysis. These devices provide direct access to blood vessels for medical procedures such as haemodialysis. Appropriate management is crucial to preventing complications and ensuring that treatments work properly.

1. Types of vascular access for haemodialysis
   * **Arteriovenous fistula (AVF): This is a** surgically created connection between an artery and a vein, usually in the arm. Over time, the vein dilates and strengthens, allowing repeated access for dialysis.
   * **Arteriovenous graft**: When an AVF is not possible, an arteriovenous graft can be performed. This involves implanting a synthetic tube to connect an artery to a vein.
   * **Central venous catheter (CVC):** This is inserted into a large vein, often the internal jugular vein. It is generally used as a temporary or emergency solution.

2. Insertion and maintenance
   * **Positioning** : Catheter placement requires a sterile procedure. An X-ray may be used to confirm positioning.
   * **Cleaning and disinfection**: Regular cleaning of the insertion site is essential to prevent infection. The area should be examined daily for signs of inflammation or infection.

- **Avoiding blockages** : Catheters can become blocked or clogged. To prevent this, they are regularly flushed with saline or heparin.

3. Complications and their prevention
- **Infections** : Catheters can be an entry point for bacteria. Sterility during insertion and maintenance is essential.
- **Thrombosis**: Blood clots can form around or inside the catheter, compromising its function.
- **Stenosis**: Blood vessels can narrow near the access, which can reduce the blood flow required for dialysis.
- **Bleeding**: Bleeding may occur if the catheter is damaged or if the insertion site is not properly cared for.

4. Patient education
It is vital to educate patients about :
- Correct handling of catheters to avoid infection.
- Signs of infection or complications, so you can intervene quickly.
- Precautions to take during daily activities to avoid damaging the catheter.

5. Withdrawal
The removal of a catheter must be carried out by a competent healthcare professional, taking care to prevent infection and ensuring that the area heals properly.

In summary, proper management of catheters and vascular access is essential to ensure effective treatment and prevent complications in nephrology. Patient education, the adoption of good clinical practice and regular monitoring all contribute to maximising the safety and efficacy of treatment.

Chapter 4:
COMPLICATIONS
AND EMERGENCY MANAGEMENT

Complications associated with dialysis.

Dialysis is a life-saving technique for many patients suffering from kidney failure. However, like any medical intervention, it is accompanied by risks and potential complications. Knowing what these complications are and how to prevent or treat them is essential to optimising patient care.

1. Immediate complications
   - **Hypotension**: A rapid drop in blood pressure during dialysis can lead to dizziness, nausea or fainting. It may be caused by fluids being removed too quickly during the session.
   - **Muscle cramps**: These can occur during or after dialysis, often due to loss of fluids or electrolytes.
   - **Reactions to the dialysis membrane**: Allergic reactions may occur, causing redness, itching or other symptoms.

2. Infectious complications
   - **Peritonitis**: for peritoneal dialysis, this is an infection of the abdominal cavity, often caused by bacterial contamination.
   - **Access infections**: Fistulas, grafts and catheters can become infected, requiring immediate care to avoid more serious complications.

3. Long-term complications
- **Anaemia**: Dialysis and kidney disease itself can lead to anaemia, as the diseased kidneys do not produce enough erythropoietin, a hormone that stimulates the production of red blood cells.
- **Bone diseases**: Kidney failure and dialysis can upset the balance of minerals in the body, leading to conditions such as renal osteodystrophy.
- **Left ventricular hypertrophy**: The heart may thicken because of the extra effort required to pump blood through narrow or stiff arteries, a common complication of kidney failure.
- **Neuropathy**: The accumulation of waste products in the blood can damage the nerves, causing tingling or pain in the extremities.

4. Other complications
- **Problems with acid-base and electrolyte balance**: Dialysis can sometimes lead to imbalances in electrolyte levels, such as potassium, which can be dangerous.
- **Dialysis exhaustion syndrome:** Intense fatigue that may follow dialysis sessions.
- **Dialysis-related amyloidosis**: Beta2-microglobulin proteins can accumulate in the blood of dialysis patients and be deposited in joints and tendons, causing pain and stiffness.

To minimise these complications, rigorous medical monitoring is essential. Regular blood tests, adjustments to dialysis treatment and careful monitoring of symptoms help to optimise patient care and improve their quality of life.

Hyper and hypotension.

Hyper- and hypotension are terms used to describe abnormal states of blood pressure. Both conditions can have significant clinical consequences and are often encountered in a variety of medical contexts, including nephrology.

<u>Hypotension</u>
Hypotension refers to abnormally low blood pressure.
- Causes:
    - Loss of blood, as in trauma or internal bleeding.
    - Severe dehydration due to vomiting, diarrhoea or insufficient fluid intake.
    - Drug reactions, particularly with antihypertensives.
    - Heart problems such as heart failure or arrhythmias.
    - Serious infections or septicaemia.
    - Autonomic nervous system dysfunction.
- Symptoms :
    - Dizziness or vertigo
    - Fainting spells
    - Fatigue
    - Nausea
    - Blurred vision
    - Confusion or disorientation
- Treatment :
    - Identify and treat the underlying cause.
    - Administer intravenous fluids to treat dehydration.
    - Adjust or change medication if necessary.
    - Use medication to increase blood pressure in certain situations.

Hypertension

Hypertension, commonly known as high blood pressure, is a condition in which the force of blood against the walls of the arteries is too high.

- Causes:
    - Genetic or hereditary factors.
    - Sedentary lifestyle.
    - High-salt diet.
    - Obesity.
    - Excessive consumption of alcohol or tobacco.
    - Certain medical conditions, such as polycystic ovary syndrome, diabetes or kidney disease.
- Symptoms :
    - Often, there are no visible symptoms, hence its nickname of "silent killer".
    - Headaches
    - Dizziness
    - Ringing in the ears
    - Visual blur
    - Shortness of breath
- Treatment :
    - Antihypertensive drugs.
    - Lifestyle changes, such as a healthy diet, regular exercise and limiting alcohol consumption.
    - Reduce your salt intake.
    - Monitor blood pressure regularly.

Hyper- and hypotension are two opposing states of blood pressure that can have serious clinical implications if not properly managed. Early recognition, regular monitoring and adaptation of treatment are essential to prevent complications associated with these conditions.

Electrolyte disorders.

Electrolyte disorders refer to an imbalance in electrolyte levels in the body. Electrolytes are essential minerals found in blood and other body fluids that conduct electricity and are essential for the normal functioning of many bodily functions. In the context of nephrology, these imbalances are particularly relevant, as the kidneys play a central role in regulating electrolyte levels.

1. Hyperkalaemia (high potassium levels)
   * Causes:
       * Renal insufficiency
       * Medications (e.g. angiotensin-converting enzyme inhibitors or non-steroidal anti-inflammatory drugs)
       * Tissue destruction (burns, trauma)
       * Metabolic acidosis
   * Symptoms :
       * Muscle weakness or paralysis
       * Cardiac arrhythmias
       * Fatigue
       * Shortness of breath
       * Palpitations
   * Treatment :
       * Medicines to stabilise the cell membrane (such as calcium gluconate)
       * Medicines to remove potassium from the body (such as cation exchange resins)
       * Dialysis

2. Hyponatremia (low sodium levels)
   * Causes:
       * Heart failure
       * Cirrhosis
       * Renal insufficiency

- Inappropriate antidiuretic secretion syndrome (SIADH)
- Symptoms :
    - Nausea and vomiting
    - Headaches
    - Fatigue
    - Convulsions
    - Coma
- Treatment :
    - Water restriction
    - Administration of saline solution
    - Medications (such as tolvaptan)

3. Hypercalcaemia (high calcium levels)
- Causes:
    - Hyperparathyroidism
    - Cancers
    - Excess vitamin D
- Symptoms :
    - Excessive thirst and frequent urination
    - Nausea and vomiting
    - Constipation
    - Muscle weakness
    - Confusion or dementia
- Treatment :
    - Intravenous hydration
    - Diuretics
    - Medications (such as bisphosphonates)

4. Hypocalcaemia (low calcium levels)
- Causes:
    - Hypoparathyroidism
    - Chronic renal failure
    - Low vitamin D intake
    - Pancreatitis
- Symptoms :
    - Tetany (involuntary muscle contractions)
    - Numbness and tingling around the mouth or in the extremities

- Muscle spasms
- Convulsions
- Treatment :
  - Calcium and vitamin D supplementation
  - Treating the underlying cause

Electrolyte imbalances can have serious effects on many body systems, particularly the heart, muscles and nervous system. Their management requires careful assessment and monitoring, as well as targeted interventions to restore balance. The kidneys play a crucial role in this regulation, hence the importance of sound nephrology in treating and preventing these imbalances.

Infection management.

Infection management is a crucial aspect of nephrology, particularly as patients with kidney disease are often immunosuppressed, either because of their underlying disease or because of the treatments they receive, especially dialysis. In addition, devices used in nephrology, such as catheters, can introduce entry points for infections. Addressing infection management in nephrology requires a comprehensive approach that encompasses prevention, diagnosis, treatment and monitoring.

1. Infection prevention
   - **Hand hygiene**: This is the simplest and most effective way of preventing infections.
   - **Sterile catheter care**: Ensure that all catheters are inserted, maintained and removed under sterile conditions.
   - **Vaccination**: Vaccinations against influenza, pneumonia and other relevant infections should be recommended.

- **Patient education**: Patients should be trained to recognise the signs of infection and to carry out appropriate home care, particularly if they are on peritoneal dialysis.

2. Identification and diagnosis
- **Symptoms to watch out for**: Fever, chills, redness or tenderness around a catheter site, cloudy or foul-smelling urine, or any other sign of infection.
- **Diagnostic tests**: Cultures of blood, urine or any peritoneal fluid to identify the pathogen. Imaging tests may also be useful.

3. Treatment
- **Antibiotics**: The choice of antibiotic will depend on the pathogen identified and its sensitivity. In some cases, empirical treatment may be started while waiting for culture results.
- **Catheter care**: In the case of catheter-related infections, the catheter may require removal, replacement or specific treatment.
- **Treatment of complications**: Infections can sometimes lead to complications such as sepsis, which require intensive management.

4. Monitoring
- **Regular monitoring**: Patients should be monitored regularly to ensure that the infection has resolved and to detect any recurrence.
- **Resistance monitoring**: In the hospital context, monitoring antibiotic-resistant strains is essential to guide future therapies.

Managing infections in nephrology is a constant challenge, requiring vigilance, training and collaboration between healthcare professionals. It is a matter of both prevention and rapid, effective treatment when infections do occur. A proactive approach can go a long way towards improving outcomes for nephrology patients and reducing the burden of nosocomial infections.

Chapter 5:
THE RELATIONSHIP WITH THE PATIENT

Effective communication
with the patient and family.

Communication is an essential pillar of healthcare. In nephrology, where patients can be faced with complex diagnoses, long-term treatments and important medical decisions, clear, compassionate and effective communication is vital. This includes not only the patient, but also their family and loved ones, who often play a crucial role in providing support and care.

1. Active listening
   - **Welcoming feelings** : Acknowledging and validating the emotions of the patient and their family. Reassure them that their concerns are heard and taken into account.
   - **Ask open-ended questions**: This gives a complete picture of the patient's situation, concerns and needs.
   - **Avoid interruptions**: Allow the patient and family to fully express their thoughts without being interrupted.

2. Clear and accessible information
   - **Simple language**: Avoid medical jargon and explain complex terms in an understandable way.
   - **Providing written resources**: Brochures, videos or websites can be useful for patients and families who want to learn more.
   - **Repeating information**: This ensures that the patient and family have understood and remembered the important details.

3. Empathetic communication
- **Validation**: Recognising the value of the feelings and experiences of patients and their families.
- **Empathy**: Putting yourself in the patient's shoes to understand their fears, hopes and needs.
- **Reassurance**: Providing emotional support, especially when difficult diagnoses are announced or major medical decisions are discussed.

4. Collaboration and shared decision-making
- **Involving the patient**: Considering the patient as a partner in medical decision-making.
- **Exploring options**: Discuss the advantages, disadvantages and possible alternatives for each therapeutic decision.
- **Respecting values and preferences**: Taking cultural, religious or personal beliefs into account in the decision-making process.

5. Managing difficult situations
- **De-escalating tension**: If a patient or family member is angry or frustrated, adopt a calm, non-defensive approach.
- **Ask for support**: Call on colleagues, social workers or psychologists if necessary.
- **Setting clear limits**: In situations where the patient or family is difficult or uncooperative, it is important to set limits while remaining respectful.

6. Confidentiality
- **Protecting information**: Ensure the confidentiality of patients' medical information, and only share it with their consent.
- **Discussion in a private environment**: Avoid discussing sensitive medical details in public or open places.

Effective communication is much more than simply exchanging information. It is an art that requires sensitivity, patience, clarity and empathy. In nephrology, where patients often face major challenges, solid communication can make the difference between confusion and clarity, isolation and support, fear and trust.

The importance of patient education.

Patient education in nephrology is a fundamental aspect that directly influences clinical outcomes, quality of life and adherence to treatment. Patients with kidney disease face a multitude of medical challenges and often have to make complex decisions about their health. Appropriate education not only enables them to better understand their disease, but also to become active and informed players in their own management.

1. Autonomy and empowerment
   - **Self-management**: Educated patients have a better ability to manage their condition, whether in terms of diet, medication management or routine care.
   - **Informed decision-making**: When they understand the ins and outs of their disease, patients are better able to make informed decisions about their treatment, whether dialysis, transplant or other interventions.

2. Better adherence to treatment
   - **Understanding medicines**: Knowing why and how to take your medication is essential to avoid complications and maximise the effectiveness of your treatment.
   - **Symptom recognition**: By knowing the common signs and symptoms of complications or deterioration

in their condition, patients can intervene more quickly or seek help when needed.

3. Reducing complications and hospital admissions
- **Avoiding mistakes**: A better understanding of prescribed treatments and diets can help prevent mistakes, such as overdosing on medication or making the wrong food choices.
- **Early detection**: Educated patients can quickly recognise the warning signs of serious complications, which can lead to faster intervention and potentially save lives.

4. Improved quality of life
- **Less anxiety**: Understanding your illness and its treatment can reduce fear and uncertainty, factors often associated with anxiety.
- **Social support**: Patients who are well informed are better able to communicate their needs and concerns to those close to them, thereby strengthening support networks.

5. Health promotion and prevention
- **Adopting a healthy lifestyle**: With the right information, patients can make informed choices about their diet, physical activity and other lifestyle habits that directly influence their kidney health.
- **Vaccination and infection prevention**: Education can emphasise the importance of regular vaccination and infection control measures, which are essential for nephrology patients.

Patient education in nephrology is a cornerstone of holistic, patient-centred care. It is a dynamic process that requires regular adjustments as the patient's condition evolves or new information becomes available. By investing in patient education, healthcare professionals can hope not only to improve clinical outcomes, but also to enrich their patients' quality of life, equipping them with the tools they need to navigate the complex landscape of nephrology with confidence.

Managing anxiety and patient stress.

Managing anxiety and stress is a critical aspect of caring for nephrology patients. Confronted with often difficult diagnoses, invasive treatments and uncertainty about the future, these patients can experience high levels of psychological distress. Adequate management of this distress is not only essential for the patient's psychological well-being, but also has a positive impact on clinical outcomes and adherence to treatment.

1. Recognition and assessment
   - **Regular screening**: Early identification of signs of anxiety and stress allows for more rapid intervention. Validated assessment tools can be used to regularly assess the patient's psychological state.
   - **Open discussion**: Fostering an environment where patients feel comfortable sharing their concerns and feelings is essential.

2. Intervention techniques
   - **Cognitive behavioural therapy (CBT)**: This approach focuses on identifying and restructuring negative thoughts and behavioural patterns. It has been shown to be effective in managing anxiety and stress.
   - **Relaxation and meditation**: Regular practice of deep relaxation techniques, such as deep breathing, meditation and visualisation, can help reduce stress levels.

3. Pharmacological support
- **Anxiolytic medication**: For some patients, medication may be necessary to manage their anxiety, especially when it is severe or persistent. However, it is crucial to monitor drug interactions, especially in renal patients.
- **Psychiatric consultation**: In serious or complex cases, a specialist consultation may be required.

4. Emotional and social support
- **Support groups**: Sharing experiences with other patients in similar situations can offer a reassuring perspective.
- **Family counselling**: Kidney disease affects the whole family. Family support and counselling can help manage collective stress.

5. Education and information
- **Reducing uncertainty**: One of the main sources of anxiety is uncertainty. Providing clear, understandable information about the disease, treatment and expectations can help reduce this feeling.
- **Workshops and seminars**: Organising educational sessions on stress and anxiety management can give patients the tools they need to cope with their condition.

6. Physical activities and leisure
- **Regular exercise**: Physical activity has proven beneficial effects on reducing stress and anxiety.
- **Therapeutic leisure**: Encouraging patients to take part in activities they enjoy, such as music, art or reading, can provide a welcome escape and distraction.

Managing anxiety and stress in nephrology patients is a crucial component of their overall care. Recognising and dealing with these emotions is not just a matter of comfort or emotional well-being; it can have a direct impact on treatment adherence, quality of life and clinical outcomes. By integrating sound psychological management into each patient's care plan, we ensure that not only their physiological needs but also their emotional and psychological needs are met.

Chapter 6:
THE WELL-BEING OF THE NURSE

Emotional and psychological challenges.

A nephrology patient's journey is littered with emotional and psychological challenges. From the diagnosis to the day-to-day management of the disease, the psychological dimension is a central pillar of the patient experience. Understanding and anticipating them enables healthcare professionals to offer holistic care, where mental well-being is just as much a priority as physical health.

1. Announcing the diagnosis
   - **Shock and denial**: The announcement of chronic kidney disease is often experienced as an upheaval, which can lead to initial denial and even incomprehension.
   - **Fear of the future**: The diagnosis is accompanied by uncertainty about the future, the course of the disease and future quality of life.

2. Modification of body image
   - **Physical changes**: Dialysis, catheters and other procedures can alter physical appearance, influencing self-perception.
   - **Self-esteem**: Dietary restrictions, fatigue or other symptoms can lead to feelings of inferiority or difference.

3. Daily treatment pressure
   - **The constraints of dialysis**: Regular dialysis sessions can feel like a constraint, encroaching on freedom and spontaneity.

- **Managing medication**: Taking and adjusting medication on a regular basis can cause stress and anxiety.

4. Fear of complications
- **Anticipating crises**: The fear of sudden complications or a deterioration in health can be omnipresent.
- **Fear of dependency**: The fear of becoming dependent on loved ones or the medical system is a common feeling.

5. Social impact
- **Isolation**: The constraints of treatment can reduce social interaction, leading to feelings of isolation or loneliness.
- **Family role**: The change in role within the family, sometimes from provider to dependent, can be difficult to accept.

6. Financial concerns
- **Treatment costs**: Even with good medical cover, the costs associated with dealing with illness can be a source of stress.
- **Professional disruption**: Illness may lead to absence from work or changes in profession, with financial implications.

7. Issues relating to transplantation
- **Waiting** : Waiting for an organ donation is a time of anxiety, hope and uncertainty.
- **Post-transplant adaptation**: Even after a successful transplant, there is a phase of adaptation with new medical routines.

8. Anticipating the end of life
  • **Existential questions**: The confrontation with mortality can give rise to profound reflections on the meaning of life, spirituality and religion.
  • **Planning**: The need to think about advance care planning or advance directives can be a source of anxiety.

The trajectory of a nephrology patient is not only marked by physical challenges; it is also deeply tinged with emotions, questions and psychological challenges. These aspects deserve just as much attention as the medical treatments. Recognising, understanding and supporting these emotional challenges is the key to truly patient-centred care, where humanity and medicine move forward hand in hand.

The importance of self-care.

Self-care, a concept that encompasses the individual activities involved in taking care of one's physical, mental and emotional health, is of paramount importance, particularly in the context of nephrology. For nurses and patients alike, self-care is much more than just a set of practices: it is a philosophy that helps to preserve integrity, strengthen resilience in the face of challenges and improve overall quality of life.

1. Self-care for the nurse
  • **Preventing burnout**: The often frenetic pace of nephrology, with its emergencies and critical issues, can quickly lead to burnout. Regular moments of self-care can help prevent this.
  • **Maintaining emotional competence**: Managing emotions, both your own and those of patients, is

fundamental. Self-care practices such as meditation and reflection help to develop better emotional regulation.

- **Perspective and balance**: By taking time for themselves, nurses can put the challenges of everyday life into perspective, renew their motivation and maintain a balance between their professional and personal lives.

2. Self-care for the patient
- **Empowerment**: Self-care enables patients to regain control over their lives and not feel solely dependent on the medical system. They become active players in their own health.
- **Symptom management**: Certain self-care practices, such as a suitable diet or relaxation, can help to reduce symptoms and even improve pain management.
- **Improved quality of life**: By regularly taking part in activities they enjoy, patients can enrich their daily lives, reduce stress and increase their general well-being.

3. How to integrate self-care
- **Education and awareness**: It is vital to provide information on the importance and benefits of self-care. Workshops, seminars or information materials can be offered.
- **Creating a self-care plan**: Everyone, whether carer or patient, should develop a self-care plan tailored to their needs and pace of life.
- **Inclusion in the care plan**: For patients, self-care can be integrated into the overall care plan, ensuring that it is considered in the same way as other medical interventions.

4. The different facets of self-care
  - **Physical**: This includes physical activity, a balanced diet, sufficient sleep and taking regular medication.
  - **Emotional**: This involves recognising, expressing and managing emotions. This can be done through journaling, therapy, relaxation or meditation.
  - **Mental**: Activities that stimulate the mind, such as reading, playing games or learning new things, contribute to mental self-care.
  - **Spiritual**: For some people, spirituality, whether religious or not, is a source of peace and meaning. This may include prayer, meditation or connecting with nature.

In the vast landscape of nephrology, where clinical and emotional challenges abound, self-care is emerging as a beacon, guiding both carers and patients towards renewed balance and well-being. Over and above a series of actions, it is a culture of kindness towards oneself that needs to be adopted and promoted. To weather the storms of kidney disease and clinical responsibilities, this practice of self-care is not a luxury, but an imperative necessity.

Striking a balance between professional and personal life.

Striking a balance between professional and personal life is a delicate dance that many professionals, including nephrology nurses, seek to master. As the hands of the clock continue to tick, these healthcare professionals try to juggle the vital care they provide to their patients with their own human needs for privacy, rest and leisure.

Imagine the beating heart of the hospital, where every tick of the clock is a life, a story, a responsibility. Nephrology nurses are immersed in this maelstrom every day, bringing comfort and care to patients with kidney disease. These moments are often tinged with strong emotions, ranging from the joy of a successful kidney transplant to the melancholy of a difficult dialysis. In this whirlwind, how can you find the time to breathe, to live, to love and to be yourself?

First of all, it is imperative to recognise the value of balance. A nurse who is exhausted, both emotionally and physically, can hardly provide optimal care. Like oxygen in a plane in distress, you have to save yourself first before you can save others.

So nurses, like so many others, need to set aside sacred moments, those bubbles of time where we disconnect from the professional and anchor ourselves in the personal. This could be an evening spent reading a book, a weekend in the countryside, or simply a few hours stolen away for a walk.

But balance isn't just about big gestures. It also lies in the small routines of everyday life. Perhaps it's taking the time to enjoy a coffee before the start of a shift, or finding a few minutes to meditate between patients. These moments, however brief, can provide a much-needed breath of fresh air.

Communication is also key. Colleagues, friends and family can offer invaluable support. They can remind nurses of the importance of taking care of themselves, offer a shoulder to lean on or simply listen.

Finding that balance is a journey, not a destination. Every day offers its share of challenges and rewards. But in this quest, it is essential to remember that to be the best in your profession, you must also be the best for yourself. So, by dancing between professional responsibilities and personal joys, nephrology nurses can not only brighten their patients' lives, but their own as well.

Chapter 7:
TESTIMONIALS AND CASE STUDIES

Typical days:
testimonials from experienced nurses.

It's often said that the best way to understand someone's day-to-day life is to walk in their shoes, even if only for a day. Nephrology, with its complexities and nuances, is no exception. What better way to paint this picture than to hear the stories of those on the front line? Here are a few testimonials from experienced nurses describing their typical days in nephrology.

1. Clara, 7 years' experience in haemodialysis
"I start my day at 6.30am. After a quick review of the files, I make sure that all the machines are ready. When the patients arrive, every minute counts. Some are frightened, others tired. My job is to alleviate their worries while ensuring their safety during dialysis. There are always complications to deal with, whether it's low blood pressure or a machine alarm. But, despite the pressure, nothing beats the satisfaction of seeing a patient leave the centre with a smile on their face."

2. Jérôme, 10 years' experience in a nephrology intensive care unit
"My service is unpredictable. I can start the day calmly, then everything changes in an instant with an emergency. The cases are often complex. There are moments of intense concentration, like when I'm fitting a catheter, but also moments of profound humanity, when I'm holding the hand of an anxious patient. Teamwork is crucial here. We are each other's eyes and ears."

3. Isabelle, 12 years' experience in therapeutic education

"My day is a mixture of teaching and listening. I inform patients about their illnesses, treatments and diets. But more often than not, I listen. The diagnosis is a shock for many people. My favourite moments? When a patient comes back months later, better informed, more confident, thanking me for helping them to navigate through this storm."

4. Léa, 9 years' experience in kidney transplantation

"Every transplant is a race against time. The day often starts early, with the announcement of a compatible donor. Every stage is crucial, from patient preparation to post-operative monitoring. The fatigue is real, but when a patient tells me they feel alive again thanks to their new kidney, it's all worth it."

These stories, though varied, share a common thread: a passion for their profession, the importance of human contact and the desire to make a difference. For these nurses, every day is both a challenge and an opportunity. They are the unsung heroes of nephrology, bringing skill, compassion and dedication at every turn.

Lessons from complex cases.

Nephrology is a field that offers a multitude of clinical situations, ranging from the simple and routine to the extraordinary and complex. The latter, with their unique challenges, often provide invaluable lessons, not only in clinical skills, but also in communication, empathy and ethics. Here are a few lessons from complex cases that have marked the careers of several nephrology professionals.

1. Communication transcends words

Case: A deaf and dumb patient regularly attended dialysis sessions. Communication was initially difficult, leading to stress and misunderstandings.

Lesson: The teams had to develop new non-verbal communication skills, use technology and be creative. The situation reminded everyone of the importance of adaptive communication and the very essence of empathy.

2. Every patient is unique, as is their treatment

Case: A patient had severe allergic reactions to drugs commonly used in dialysis, making the process dangerous for her.

Lesson: Standard protocols had to be adapted to meet the needs of this patient. This highlighted the need for an individualised approach to care and the flexibility required to deal with atypical situations.

3. Ethics at the heart of decision-making

Case: A patient with end-stage renal disease and strict religious beliefs was refusing a potential transplant. The medical team was torn between respecting his choices and offering him the best possible quality of life.

Lesson: Respect for patient autonomy is paramount, even if it runs counter to the personal beliefs of the carer. Ethical decision-making requires open discussion, patient participation and sometimes the support of an ethics committee.

4. Resilience in the face of the unexpected

Case: Following a major power cut in a dialysis unit, many patients were unable to receive their treatment, putting their lives at risk.

Lesson: The ability to adapt and react quickly is essential. The teams had to organise transport to other centres, reprioritise cases and communicate effectively with patients and families. This reinforced the importance of emergency preparedness and team cohesion.

5. Technology is a tool, not a solution

Case: A patient was using a telemedicine device for his home dialysis sessions. Although technically everything was working, the patient felt isolated and anxious.

Lesson: Technology can improve the efficiency of care, but it cannot replace the human touch. Regular follow-up, understanding patients' emotional needs and offering holistic support are essential.

These cases, among many others, illustrate the richness and complexity of nephrology. They serve as a reminder that, although each situation is unique, the lessons learnt have universal application, enriching clinical practice and strengthening the bond between carer and cared-for.

Inspiration and motivation to continue along this path.

Nephrology nurses, like many healthcare professionals, can sometimes feel tired, weary or even hopeless in the face of daily challenges. Yet there are always things that drive them to persevere, stay committed and continue to provide quality care. Here are a few sources of inspiration and motivation that encourage these dedicated professionals to keep going:

1. Therapeutic successes

There is nothing more gratifying for a nephrology nurse than to see a patient blossom after a successful transplant or to see a tangible improvement in quality of life thanks to effective dialysis. These medical successes are a reminder of the direct impact of their work.

2. Patient-caregiver relationships

Over time, nurses develop strong bonds with their patients. These relationships, built on trust and compassion, often become a source of inspiration. Seeing a patient overcome obstacles, thanks in part to the nurse's help and support, reinforces the sense of duty.

3. Constant learning
Medicine is constantly evolving, and nephrology is no exception. New research, techniques and technologies provide opportunities for learning and innovation. This constant quest for knowledge renews the passion of many professionals.

4. Community impact
Nurses don't just work on an individual level; their work has an impact on the whole community. By educating patients and promoting awareness of kidney health, they play an essential role in preventing and managing kidney disease at community level.

5. Peer support
Working as part of a multidisciplinary team offers the opportunity to support each other and share experiences and challenges. Knowing that they are not alone, that their colleagues share the same difficulties and successes, is an undeniable source of motivation.

6. Inspiring stories
Every patient has a story, and sometimes it's that story that inspires the most. Whether it's someone who has overcome enormous obstacles to lead a normal life thanks to dialysis, or an organ donor who has given someone a second chance, these stories reinforce the profound meaning of their vocation.

7. Personal commitment
Many nurses remember why they chose this profession. For some, it was a personal vocation born of personal or family experience of kidney disease. For others, it's a

passion for care, science and humanity. Reconnecting with this initial source of inspiration can rekindle the flame.

The path of the nephrology nurse is not without its challenges, but it is precisely these challenges that make the profession so rewarding. By continually reminding themselves of what motivates them, these professionals find the strength and inspiration to move forward and continue to make a difference.

Chapter 8:
ETHICS AND NEPHROLOGY

Common ethical dilemmas
in nephrology.

Nephrology, like many other medical specialities, is faced with complex ethical dilemmas. These dilemmas often arise when fundamental ethical principles come into conflict. Here are some common ethical dilemmas faced by nephrology professionals:

1. Autonomy vs. benevolence
   - *Situation*: A patient refuses a kidney transplant that could potentially prolong his life.
   - *Dilemma*: Respect the patient's choice (autonomy) or persuade them to accept the treatment that is in their best interests (beneficence)?

2. Rationing resources
   - *The situation*: Resources for dialysis are limited, and decisions need to be made about who will be prioritised for treatment.
   - *Dilemma*: How can we allocate limited resources fairly while respecting the intrinsic value of each life?

3. Life vs. quality of life
   - *Situation*: An elderly patient suffering from several co-morbidities has little chance of long-term survival, even with dialysis.
   - *Dilemma*: Should we continue intensive treatment to prolong life, or focus on the patient's comfort and quality of life?

4. Informed consent in the context of culture and religion
   - *Situation*: A patient refuses treatment because of his religious beliefs, even if this puts his life at risk.
   - *Dilemma*: How can we respect patients' cultural and religious beliefs while ensuring their health and safety?

5. Transplants and selection criteria
   - *Situation*: Two patients need a transplant, but only one organ is available.
   - *Dilemma*: How do we decide who should receive the organ? Should the decision be based on age, compatibility, waiting time or other criteria?

6. Confidentiality vs. duty to warn
   - *Situation*: A dialysis patient admits that he is not adhering properly to his treatment or that he is using banned substances, which could put him at risk.
   - *Dilemma*: How do you balance respect for patient confidentiality with the duty to prevent danger?

7. End of life and cessation of treatment
   - *Situation*: A patient with end-stage renal disease asks to be taken off dialysis.
   - *Dilemma*: How can we meet this demand while ensuring that patients are fully informed and not subject to external pressure?

Ethical dilemmas in nephrology highlight the importance of sound ethical training and professional support for healthcare professionals. They also show the need for multidisciplinary approaches, where doctors, nurses, social workers, ethicists and other specialists work together to find the best solutions for patients.

Informed consent and patients' rights.

Informed consent is not just an administrative formality. It is a fundamental pillar of modern medical care, reflecting a profound respect for the rights and dignity of the patient. The underlying idea is that every individual has inherent autonomy, and as such should have a determining voice in decisions about their own health.

In the world of nephrology, the path to treatment is often complex. Whether it's the prospect of dialysis, kidney transplantation or other interventions, patients are often faced with a myriad of choices. Each option has its own benefits, risks and long-term implications. This is where informed consent comes in.

The process begins with open communication between the healthcare professional and the patient. Instead of simply prescribing a solution, the doctor or nurse presents each available option, detailing the expected benefits, potential risks and possible alternatives. However, this is not simply a matter of providing an avalanche of medical information. The information must be given in an understandable way, taking into account the patient's level of knowledge and concerns.

But informed consent goes far beyond simple understanding. Patients must also have the freedom to make a choice. This means that they should feel no pressure, whether from medical staff, family or anyone else. Their decision, whether in favour of or against a proposed treatment, must be respected. After all, it is the patient who will experience the direct consequences of this decision.

Patients' rights are intrinsically linked to the concept of informed consent. Every patient has the right to know, the right to ask questions and, above all, the right to refuse treatment. This approach places the patient at the centre of medical care, recognising him or her as a major player in his or her own health, and not simply as a passive recipient of care.

Informed consent and patient rights strengthen the bond of trust between patient and healthcare professional. In a speciality as complex as nephrology, this trust is invaluable. It ensures that, whatever route is chosen, the patient and the healthcare professional move forward together, in a partnership based on mutual respect, understanding and commitment.

End of life and palliative care in nephrology.

The end of life in nephrology is a deeply emotional and often complex subject. While medical advances have made it possible to prolong the lives of many people with kidney disease, there comes a time when quality of life can be seriously compromised. This is when palliative care comes into its own.

Palliative care in nephrology aims to improve the quality of life of patients and their families in the face of the consequences of advanced kidney disease. Contrary to what you might think, it does not focus solely on the last days or weeks of life. They intervene as soon as severe kidney disease is diagnosed, offering care focused on relieving pain and other troublesome symptoms, and providing psychological, social and spiritual support.

In nephrology, the introduction of palliative care can be complex. The patient may have been on dialysis for years, battling the associated complications on a daily basis. The decision to stop or not to start dialysis is a difficult one, and needs to be discussed with the patient, their family and the medical team. It requires a thorough assessment of the potential benefits of continuing dialysis in terms of the patient's quality of life and comfort.

One of the fundamental aspects of palliative care is dialogue. It is essential that the patient, family and medical team communicate openly about expectations, concerns and hopes. These conversations can be difficult, touching on issues such as advance directives, refusing or stopping treatment, and wishes for the last moments of life. Yet it is through these sincere discussions that we can ensure a peaceful and dignified end to life.

Another key element of palliative care is the multidisciplinary approach. The team may include not only nephrologists, but also specialist palliative care nurses, psychologists, social workers, chaplains and other professionals. Each brings their own expertise, ensuring that all the patient's needs, whether physical, emotional, social or spiritual, are taken into account.

The end of life in nephrology can be marked by pain, exhaustion and distress, both for the patient and his or her family. Palliative care aims to ease these burdens, offer comfort and ensure that each day, however difficult, is lived with dignity and respect. While death is an inevitable reality, how we approach it can make all the difference, and nephrology palliative care reminds us that every moment counts.

Chapter 9:
CULTURE
AND DIVERSITY IN NEPHROLOGY

The challenges of care patients from a wide range of backgrounds.

Caring for patients from diverse backgrounds presents a unique set of challenges for healthcare professionals, particularly in a field as complex as nephrology. Cultural, socio-economic, linguistic and religious diversity can have a profound impact on the way patients perceive their illness, their treatment and the relationship with their medical team.

One of the first challenges is the language barrier. For a patient who does not speak the same language as their carer, understanding the subtleties of a diagnosis or medical procedure can be tricky. It is therefore vital to have access to qualified medical interpreters who can translate not only the words, but also the nuances and underlying implications.

Cultural differences can also influence how a patient perceives their illness and its treatment. For example, some cultures may have specific beliefs about the causes of illness or strong opinions about Western treatments. For these patients, the integration of traditional medicines or spiritual practices may be essential to their well-being.

Socio-economic challenges also play a major role. Patients from disadvantaged backgrounds may find it difficult to access care, follow treatment or adopt healthy lifestyles due to financial constraints or lack of adequate resources. In addition, the stigma associated with certain illnesses or poverty may prevent these patients from actively seeking medical help.

Religious beliefs and practices can also influence a patient's approach to treatment. For example, some patients may refuse blood transfusions or organ transplants for religious reasons. In such cases, it is crucial that the medical team is informed and respectful of these beliefs while seeking alternative solutions to ensure the best possible care.

The solution to these challenges lies in the cultural training of healthcare professionals. This involves not only knowledge of different cultures and traditions, but also the ability to listen actively and interact with empathy and open-mindedness.

It is also essential to have a diverse team capable of understanding and responding to the unique needs of each patient. Collaboration with community leaders, cultural health experts and patient associations can also prove invaluable.

The challenge of caring for patients from diverse backgrounds is not just to treat a kidney disease, but to understand and respect the whole person, with all their particularities, beliefs and experiences. It is this holistic approach that guarantees high-quality care and builds trust between the patient and his or her medical team.

The importance of cultural sensitivity.

Cultural sensitivity in the medical field, and in nephrology in particular, is much more than mere convenience. It is an essential pillar of effective, empathetic and respectful medical care. At a time when we live in a globalised world, when more and more patients from different backgrounds are coming together in healthcare establishments, recognising and valuing this diversity is not just a moral act, but also a clinical imperative.

Firstly, cultural sensitivity contributes to better communication. When medical staff are able to recognise and understand linguistic and cultural differences, they are better able to provide clear information, thus avoiding misunderstandings that could be detrimental to patient care. This extends beyond language to understanding non-verbal expressions, beliefs about health and illness, and family and community values.

Secondly, being sensitive to cultural differences helps to build a relationship of trust. Mistrust of the medical system is a real barrier for many patients, often rooted in negative past experiences, stereotypes or cultural beliefs. By treating each patient as a unique individual and valuing their culture, healthcare professionals can create an environment in which patients feel respected, listened to and understood.

Cultural sensitivity also helps to improve the quality of care by ensuring that the treatments offered are appropriate and effective. Some communities may be at greater risk of certain diseases or have different responses to certain treatments. In addition, the way in which patients perceive and manage pain, illness or medical treatment varies greatly depending on their culture. Taking this into account ensures that the care plan is truly tailored to each individual.

Finally, cultural sensitivity helps to reduce health inequalities. Cultural barriers can often lead to delayed diagnosis, poor adherence to treatment or a lack of prevention. By being sensitive to the specific needs of each community, healthcare professionals can help to bridge these gaps and offer equitable care to all.

Cultural sensitivity is not simply an additional skill, but an essential component of modern medicine. It enriches the relationship between patient and carer, improves the quality of care and reinforces medical ethics based on respect, empathy and fairness. As such, ongoing training and development in cultural sensitivity should be at the heart of medical education programmes and health policies.

Ethnic characteristics kidney disease.

Like many other diseases, kidney disease does not always manifest itself in the same way in all individuals. Ethnic and genetic variations can influence the prevalence, diagnosis, progression and response to treatment of kidney disease. By understanding these ethnic differences, healthcare professionals can offer more individualised and effective care.

1. Ethnic prevalence:
   - **African-Americans and Afro-Caribbeans**: These populations have a higher prevalence of chronic kidney disease, particularly segmental and focal glomerulosclerosis. The APOL1 gene is particularly implicated, conferring an increased risk of kidney disease in individuals with two copies of certain variants.
   - **Asians**: Some Asian groups, particularly those of South Asian origin, have a higher prevalence of diabetes, which is a major risk factor for kidney disease.

- **Hispanics and Latin Americans**: Although they have a higher risk of diabetes, they appear to have a lower risk of progression to end-stage renal disease than non-Hispanics.

2. Treatment response and management:
   - Some drugs, such as ACE inhibitors or angiotensin receptor antagonists, may be more or less effective depending on ethnic origin. For example, African-Americans sometimes respond less well to these treatments than non-Hispanic whites.

3. Genetic aspects:
   - Specific mutations, such as the APOL1 gene mentioned above, may predispose certain ethnic populations to kidney disease. Identifying these genetic variations will provide a better understanding of the disease and could point the way to targeted therapeutic approaches.

4. Social and cultural factors:
   - Perceptions of illness, adherence to treatment and access to care may vary between ethnic groups due to cultural, socio-economic or linguistic factors. For example, some patients may prefer traditional remedies or have specific beliefs about the cause of their illness.

5. Diagnosis and progression:
   - Standardised diagnostic criteria, such as serum creatinine levels to assess renal function, may need to be adjusted for ethnicity, as reference levels may vary between groups.

6. Associated problems:
   - Certain ethnic groups may have more frequent co-morbidities, such as hypertension or diabetes, which have a direct influence on kidney disease.

A patient's ethnic origin plays a significant role in the manifestation and management of kidney disease. Clinicians need to be aware of these particularities in order to offer optimal management. An individualised approach, taking account of ethnic and cultural diversity, is essential for precision medicine in the field of nephrology.

Chapter 10:
TECHNOLOGY AND INNOVATION IN NEPHROLOGY

New technologies in dialysis.

The rapid development of medical technology has had a major impact on the field of dialysis. These advances aim to improve the effectiveness of treatment, reduce associated complications and offer patients a better quality of life. Here's an overview of new technologies in dialysis and how they are transforming the nephrology landscape.

1. New-generation dialysis machines:
   - These modern devices offer greater precision in fluid control, enabling better elimination of waste products and more precise electrolyte balance.
   - They feature intuitive touch screens, improved user interfaces and easy integration with hospital information systems.

2. Portable dialysis:
   - The advent of portable dialysis machines means that patients can receive their treatment in the comfort of their own home. This can reduce the stress associated with frequent visits to the centre and offer greater flexibility.
   - These devices are smaller, lighter and easier to use.

3. Needle-free dialysis:
   - Research is underway to develop dialysis systems that do not use needles, thereby reducing pain and the risk of infection.

4. Telemedicine:

- With the integration of communication technologies, patients can now have consultations with their nephrologists via telemedicine platforms. This is particularly useful for patients who live far away or for follow-up consultations.

5. Artificial intelligence and data analysis:

- By using AI to analyse data from dialysis sessions, complications can be anticipated, treatment parameters optimised and treatment personalised.
- AI-based systems can also help with the early detection of infections or equipment malfunctions.

6. Improvements in dialysis membranes:

- The new membranes are designed to be more biocompatible, reducing inflammatory reactions and offering improved haemodialysis.
- Some innovative membranes enable better elimination of medium-sized molecules, which have traditionally been difficult to filter.

7. Virtual reality training:

- Healthcare professionals can now use virtual reality to train for dialysis procedures, enabling more immersive and hands-on training.

8. Research into artificial kidneys:

- Progress is being made in the development of artificial kidneys, which could offer a long-term alternative to dialysis. Although this technology is still in its infancy, it represents a glimmer of hope for the future of nephrology.

New technologies in dialysis are revolutionising the management of patients suffering from kidney failure. They offer not only improvements in the quality and effectiveness of treatment, but also a better quality of life for patients, by placing the power in their hands and actively involving them in their own care.

Digital applications and tools for patient management.

In an era dominated by digital technology, medicine is no exception. Digital tools have transformed the way medical care is delivered, making patient management more efficient, transparent and patient-centred. Here are some of the digital applications and tools that are making their mark in patient management, particularly in nephrology.

1. Electronic medical records (EMR):
   - **Description: These are** digitised databases containing all a patient's medical information.
   - **Benefits:** Ease of access, sharing of information between healthcare professionals, reduction in medical errors and better coordination of care.

2. Patient portals:
   - **Description:** Online platforms where patients can access their medical information, book appointments, renew prescriptions and communicate with their healthcare providers.
   - **Benefits:** Increases patient autonomy, improves communication and optimises administrative management.

3. Telemedicine applications:
   - **Description:** Allows remote consultations, whether by video, audio or chat.
   - **Benefits:** Increased accessibility, reduced waiting times and convenience for patients and doctors.

4. Remote monitoring applications:
- **Description:** These applications make it possible to monitor vital signs, treatment adherence and other relevant data in real time or close to it.
- **Benefits:** Early detection of complications or deviations, improved adherence to treatment and greater patient involvement.

5. Patient education platforms:
- **Description:** Websites or mobile applications that provide reliable information on diseases, treatments and preventive care.
- **Benefits:** Better informed patients, ability to make informed decisions and improved disease management.

6. Appointment management systems:
- **Description:** Tools that automate the booking, confirmation and reminder of appointments.
- **Benefits:** Reduced absence, optimised clinical time and improved patient experience.

7. Applications for medication management:
- **Description:** These applications remind patients when to take their medication, monitor drug interactions and can even be used to renew prescriptions.
- **Benefits:** Improves adherence to medication, reduces medication errors and simplifies day-to-day management.

8. Social interaction platforms:
- **Description:** Disease-specific forums, groups or social networks enabling patients to share their experiences.
- **Benefits:** Emotional support, sharing of practical advice and a sense of belonging to a community.

9. Analysis and artificial intelligence tools:
- **Description:** Use data to predict risks, advise on optimal treatments and anticipate patient needs.
- **Benefits:** More proactive care, reduced costs and improved quality of care.

10. Virtual or augmented reality applications:
- **Description:** Used for medical training, distraction during painful procedures or rehabilitation.
- **Benefits:** Innovative therapeutic approaches, greater patient involvement and improved clinical effectiveness.

These tools, combined with appropriate training of healthcare professionals and adoption by patients, have the potential to transform nephrology and other medical fields, offering more personalised, patient-centred and evidence-based care.

The future of telemedicine in nephrology.

Telemedicine, or the practice of caring for patients at a distance using communication technologies, has seen phenomenal growth in recent years. In nephrology, this approach can be particularly beneficial, given the need to monitor patients regularly, adjust their treatments and provide ongoing education. Let's take a look at what the future may hold for telemedicine in this specialist field.

1. Expansion of homecare services:
One of the main trends is the migration of care from traditional dialysis centres to the patient's home. Telemedicine is facilitating this transition by enabling remote monitoring of dialysis sessions, regular consultations with nephrologists and real-time communication with carers.

2. Self-monitoring tools:
With the development of connected devices, patients can now self-monitor essential parameters such as blood pressure, weight or electrolyte levels. This data can be automatically transmitted to healthcare professionals via secure platforms for analysis and rapid intervention if necessary.

3. Enhanced education and training:
Telemedicine offers the opportunity to hold education sessions for patients, covering topics such as medication management, dietetics, or even preparation for a kidney transplant.

4. Wider access:
For patients living in remote or underserved areas, telemedicine breaks down geographical barriers, offering easier access to specialists and quality care.

5. Interprofessional collaboration:
Telemedicine platforms promote closer collaboration between nephrologists, nurses, dieticians, social workers and other members of the care team, even if they are geographically dispersed.

6. Artificial intelligence and predictive analysis:
The future of telemedicine could incorporate more AI to analyse trends in patient data, predict potential complications and advise on the best interventions or treatment adjustments.

7. Personalised care:
Based on real-time patient data and history, telemedicine can facilitate a more personalised approach, tailoring care to each patient's specific needs.

8. Cost savings:

By avoiding unnecessary hospitalisations, complications or repeat visits, telemedicine has the potential to significantly reduce the costs associated with the management of nephrology patients.

9. Challenges ahead:

Although promising, telemedicine in nephrology will have to overcome certain challenges, such as concerns about privacy, data security, regulatory barriers, and resistance to change on the part of certain professionals or patients.

Telemedicine is set to become a major pillar of nephrology in the future. It presents a unique opportunity to rethink the way care is delivered, empower patients and optimise clinical outcomes. However, its success will depend on widespread adoption, appropriate regulation and ongoing training for healthcare professionals.

Chapter 11:
RESEARCH AND PARTICIPATION CLINICAL STUDIES

Introduction to clinical research in nephrology.

In the vast field of medicine, clinical research remains the fundamental pillar that fuels and shapes the evolution of medical care. In nephrology, a speciality devoted to kidney disease, clinical research is of vital importance in improving patients' quality of life, proposing new therapies and, ultimately, saving lives. This introduction to clinical research in nephrology aims to shed light on its role, challenges and successes.

1. The importance of clinical research in nephrology:
Nephrology, like other medical specialities, is constantly evolving. Each discovery or innovation is often the result of many years, or even decades, of clinical research. Whether it's to understand the genesis of a kidney disease, develop a new treatment or improve dialysis protocols, clinical research is at the heart of these advances.

2. Types of research in nephrology:
- **Basic research:** This seeks to understand the cellular and molecular mechanisms of kidney disease.
- **Translational research:** This bridges the gap between basic and clinical research, by applying laboratory discoveries to patient care.
- **Clinical research:** This involves trials on patients themselves, often to test new treatments, interventions or devices.

- **Epidemiological research:** This research focuses on the trends, causes and effects of health problems in specific populations.

3. Conducting a clinical trial:
The conduct of a clinical trial in nephrology follows well-defined stages, from the pre-clinical phase to phase IV, each phase having a precise objective and success criteria.

4. Challenges of clinical research in nephrology:
Despite its importance, research in nephrology faces challenges such as limited funding, ethical concerns related to patient trials, or the length of trials needed to prove the efficacy of an intervention.

5. Impact of technology:
With the advent of biotechnology, genomics and bioinformatics, nephrology research has undergone phenomenal growth. The identification of biomarkers, gene therapy and the use of artificial intelligence to predict disease are just some of the recent innovations.

6. Ethics in clinical research:
Clinical research must always be conducted in accordance with medical ethics, guaranteeing safety, autonomy, beneficence and justice for all participants.

7. International collaboration:
The global challenges of kidney health require international collaboration. Clinical research networks and consortia bring together researchers from all over the world to work on common issues.

8. The role of nurses in clinical research:
In addition to doctors and researchers, nurses play a crucial role in the conduct of clinical research, monitoring patients, administering treatments and collecting data.

Clinical research in nephrology is more than essential. It is the promise of a better future for all patients with kidney disease. Every nurse, doctor and nephrology researcher contributes, in their own way, to this brighter, more hopeful future.

The role of the nurse in clinical trials.

When we think of clinical trials, we tend to think immediately of researchers and doctors. However, nurses play an equally essential, indeed pivotal, role in the implementation, monitoring and success of these studies. Their involvement in clinical trials is multidimensional, combining clinical, administrative and interpersonal skills.

1. Patient recruitment and assessment:
Nurses are often the first healthcare professionals that patients meet when they consider taking part in a clinical trial. They are responsible for pre-selecting patients according to inclusion and exclusion criteria, and for obtaining informed consent after providing a full and comprehensible explanation of the trial.

2. Treatment administration:
Depending on the trial protocol, nurses may be responsible for administering drugs, following specific protocols or monitoring interventions. They must ensure that each step is carried out in accordance with the trial guidelines.

3. Monitoring and assessment:
Nurses play a central role in monitoring side effects and adverse reactions. They regularly assess patients' state of health, collect data and alert the medical team to any problems or concerns.

4. Data collection and documentation:

Rigour is essential in clinical trials. Nurses are often responsible for the accurate and detailed recording of data, be it vital measurements, laboratory results or any other parameter relevant to the study.

5. Education and support:

Patients enrolled in a clinical trial may have concerns or uncertainties. Nurses listen carefully, reassure patients and answer their questions throughout the study.

6. Coordination with the multidisciplinary team:

Clinical trial nurses work closely with a variety of professionals - researchers, doctors, pharmacists, laboratory technicians - ensuring smooth communication and effective coordination for the smooth running of the trial.

7. Compliance with ethical standards:

In accordance with ethical principles, nurses ensure that the rights, safety and well-being of trial participants are protected. They also ensure that the patient can withdraw from the trial at any time, without affecting the quality of care received.

8. Ongoing training:

The field of clinical trials is constantly evolving. As a result, the nurses involved must regularly update their knowledge of trial protocols, therapeutic advances and ethical guidelines.

The clinical trial nurse is an essential link, acting as a bridge between patients and the research team. Their role is complex, requiring a mix of clinical, interpersonal and organisational skills, all with the ultimate aim of improving care and treatment for future patients.

How to stay informed
the latest advances?

In today's ever-changing medical world, it is crucial for all healthcare professionals to keep up to date with new discoveries, techniques, therapies and recommendations. For nephrology nurses, this quest for knowledge is all the more relevant, given the importance of their speciality. Here are a few strategies for keeping abreast of the latest advances in the field:

1. Take part in continuing education courses:
Most medical institutions and professional associations regularly offer further training in the form of courses, workshops or seminars. These courses offer not only theoretical knowledge, but also an opportunity to discuss experiences and practices with colleagues.

2. Joining professional associations:
Professional associations, such as the Nephrology Association or the Dialysis Nurses Association, often publish newsletters, journals or magazines containing articles on the latest research, recommendations and case studies.

3. Attend conferences and symposia:
These events bring together experts from around the world to discuss recent advances, present studies and share experiences. They are also excellent places for networking and exchanging ideas.

4. Subscribe to medical journals:
Journals specialising in nephrology or nursing regularly publish research, reviews and review articles. Having access to these publications can provide valuable information.

5. Use online resources:

With increasing digitalisation, many platforms, forums and blogs dedicated to nephrology are available. They can offer webinars, online courses, discussions and even simulations to train in new techniques.

6. Establish a professional network:

Regularly exchanging with colleagues, mentors and other healthcare professionals can provide informal but valuable information on emerging trends and new practices.

7. Participating in clinical research:

Being actively involved in clinical research offers a first-hand perspective on current innovations and trial treatments.

8. Use digital applications and tools:

Dedicated nephrology apps can provide regular updates, quizzes, case studies and other educational resources.

9. Make time for monitoring:

Dedicating time specifically to reading, learning and updating knowledge is essential. This could be an hour a week or a few minutes every day.

10. Encourage a learning culture:

Fostering a culture where colleagues actively share their findings, participate in group discussions or hold briefings can benefit the whole team.

Keeping abreast of the latest advances requires a continuous and conscious effort, but the benefits in terms of quality of care, professional satisfaction and career development are inestimable. In the fast-paced, dynamic world of modern medicine, it is imperative that every healthcare professional takes the lead to ensure optimal patient care.

Chapter 12:
INTER-HOSPITAL COLLABORATION

Care coordination
with other medical specialities.

The role of a nephrology nurse often goes beyond the boundaries of their own speciality. Renal pathologies can have ramifications and interconnections with other medical disorders, requiring close collaboration with other medical specialities. This interdisciplinary synergy is essential to ensure that patients receive the best possible overall care.

1. The interdependence of body systems:
The kidneys, although distinct in function, are inextricably linked to other body systems. Whether it is the cardiovascular, endocrine or bone systems, kidney failure can have wide and varied implications. For example, chronic kidney disease can increase the risk of heart disease.

2. Interaction with cardiology:
Patients with renal failure often have cardiac comorbidities. Hypertension, common in renal patients, requires coordinated management between the nephrologist and the cardiologist. Similarly, drugs prescribed by cardiologists can affect renal function and vice versa.

3. Collaboration with endocrinology:
Hormonal imbalances, particularly in diabetic patients, can affect kidney health. Working with endocrinologists to manage and monitor glucose levels, as well as to adjust medication, is crucial.

4. Orthopaedics and bone health:
Kidney disease can impact calcium and phosphorus metabolism, leading to bone abnormalities. Close collaboration with orthopaedic surgeons and rheumatologists is often necessary.

5. Nutrition and dietetics:
The dietary needs of nephrology patients are specific. Coordination with specialist dieticians can help to develop appropriate dietary plans, thereby improving the patient's quality of life.

6. Nephro-psychiatry:
The psychological implications of kidney disease, especially in patients on dialysis, cannot be underestimated. Liaison with psychiatry or psychology is often beneficial in addressing the emotional and mental aspects of the disease.

7. Pneumology and nephrology:
Some diseases, such as lupus, can affect both the kidneys and the lungs. In these situations, interdisciplinary collaboration is essential.

The complexity of nephrology care requires a holistic vision, embracing the patient as a whole. Coordination and collaboration with other medical specialities are therefore essential. The nephrology nurse, as the linchpin of this coordination, plays an essential role in integrating and synthesising multidisciplinary care, thereby ensuring continuity and efficiency of care.

Communication
between the various health services.

Communication is the central pillar of efficient medical care. In the complex environment of hospitals and clinics, collaboration between different departments is commonplace, requiring accurate, timely and clear exchanges of information to ensure patient safety and well-being. For a nephrology nurse, this is often a balancing act, ensuring that essential information is passed on while respecting patient confidentiality.

1. The importance of interdisciplinary communication:
The complexity of kidney disease often means that patients need to be cared for by several specialists at the same time. Whether it's a cardiologist, an endocrinologist, a surgeon or a dietician, coordinating care requires fluid communication.

2. Communication tools:
Hospital information systems, electronic medical records and telecommunication platforms allow information to be shared rapidly. It is essential that nurses are comfortable using these tools to ensure that data is transmitted effectively.

3. Interdisciplinary meetings:
These regular meetings between professionals from different specialities encourage direct exchange, enabling cases to be discussed, treatment plans to be drawn up and patients to be monitored.

4. Continuity of care:
When a patient is transferred from one department to another or when their condition requires care at home, communication between departments is crucial to ensure a smooth transition and continuity of care.

5. The challenges of communication:
Despite the importance of communication, barriers can exist. Whether these are technological barriers, lack of time, medical hierarchies or differences of opinion, it is essential to be aware of these challenges and work to overcome them.

6. The role of the educator:
In addition to communicating with other professionals, the nephrology nurse often plays the role of educator. Whether it's informing another department about the specifics of nephrology or providing continuing education for their peers, the ability to communicate clearly and pedagogically is invaluable.

7. Respect for confidentiality:
All communication must respect medical confidentiality and the confidentiality of patient information. It is crucial to ensure that only the professionals directly involved in the patient's care have access to the relevant data.

In today's dynamic and interconnected medical environment, communication between departments is an essential skill for any healthcare professional. For the nephrology nurse, it ensures holistic, integrated and effective patient care, while strengthening interdisciplinary links and promoting a culture of collaboration and mutual respect.

Mentoring programmes and professional exchanges.

In today's ever-changing medical world, continuing education and the exchange of knowledge are key to ensuring optimal patient care. For nephrology nurses, mentoring and professional exchange programmes offer unique opportunities for learning, professional development and sharing experiences.

1. Mentoring: a springboard for young professionals.
Nurses starting out in nephrology can sometimes feel overwhelmed by the complexity of the specialty. Having a mentor, an experienced professional, can be a lifeline. This guide, with its wealth of experience, can help navigate the clinical, emotional and ethical challenges encountered on a daily basis.

2. The transmission of knowledge.
Mentoring doesn't just benefit the mentee. It's an opportunity for experienced nurses to pass on their knowledge, renew their passion for their specialty and contribute to the development of their profession.

3. Professional exchanges: beyond borders.
The opportunity to work or observe in another department, clinic or even country can provide a refreshing perspective. These exchange programmes enable nurses to gain a deeper understanding of best practice, innovations and different approaches to care.

4. Networking and collaboration.
These programmes encourage the creation of professional networks. The relationships established can be invaluable for exchanging information, collaborating on research projects or even obtaining advice on complex cases.

5. The challenges of adaptation.
Although professional exchanges are enriching, they can also be demanding. Adapting to a new environment, another culture or different practices can be a challenge. However, these challenges are often a source of professional and personal growth.

6. Institutional support.

Institutional support is essential for these programmes to succeed. Hospitals, clinics and professional organisations play a key role in setting up, funding and promoting these initiatives.

7. The importance of feedback.

Whether in a mentoring programme or a professional exchange, feedback is crucial. It helps to guide learning, reinforce skills and correct shortcomings.

Mentoring and professional exchanges offer nephrology nurses invaluable opportunities for learning, collaboration and professional development. In a profession where knowledge is rapidly evolving, these programmes ensure that nurses remain at the forefront of their specialty, ready to provide the best possible care to their patients.

Chapter 13:
ADMINISTRATION
AND LEADERSHIP IN NEPHROLOGY

The move towards management roles.

Every healthcare professional, particularly in the field of nephrology, starts their career with a solid technical and clinical background. However, with time, experience and a desire to contribute on a broader scale, many find themselves drawn to management roles. These positions offer a unique opportunity to shape patient care, clinical processes and even institutional culture.

1. From clinical to management:
The transition from clinical nurse to manager often requires a transition in terms of both skills and mentality. The focus is no longer just on the patient's well-being, but also on the optimal functioning of an entire unit or department.

2. Essential management skills:
In addition to clinical skills, a nurse manager will need to master human resource management, leadership, strategic planning, budget management, and data-driven decision making.

3. The challenges of transition:
Moving into a management role can be accompanied by challenges such as dealing with former colleagues, taking unpopular decisions, or the need to reconcile sometimes divergent clinical and administrative objectives.

4. Impact on patient care:
Even in a management position, the main objective

remains to improve the quality of patient care. A nurse manager can have a significant impact by optimising processes, promoting evidence-based practices and instilling a culture of patient safety.

5. Further training:
Moving into management roles often requires additional training, from short courses in leadership to a Masters in Health Administration.

6. Networking opportunities:
Management roles offer the opportunity to connect with leaders and decision-makers from diverse backgrounds, learn best practice from other institutions and contribute to the national discourse on healthcare.

7. Balancing management and clinical roles:
Some nurse managers choose to retain a clinical role, however small, in order to stay in touch with the reality on the ground, keep their skills up to date and remain credible with their team.

Moving into management roles is a rewarding path that enables nephrology nurses to have a wider impact on the healthcare system. While requiring adaptation and the acquisition of new skills, it offers the opportunity to positively influence the quality of care, patient satisfaction and the well-being of teams.

The importance of clinical leadership.

The world of healthcare is constantly evolving, with both clinical and managerial challenges multiplying. In this context, clinical leadership is emerging not only as a key skill, but also as a vital element in guiding and influencing the direction that healthcare takes. For nephrology nurses, understanding and embodying this leadership is all the more crucial.

1. Clinical leadership defined:
Unlike pure management, clinical leadership focuses on improving healthcare through clinical practice. It is about guiding, influencing and inspiring peers to promote a culture of clinical excellence.

2. Beyond technical competence:
While valuing clinical mastery, leadership goes beyond this. It encompasses the ability to collaborate, communicate effectively, solve problems and innovate for the well-being of patients.

3. The role of nurse leaders:
Nurses, because of their constant proximity to patients, are ideally placed to observe and identify areas requiring improvement. They can thus become advocates for change and promoters of innovations in care.

4. Influence on organisational culture:
A clinical leader helps to create a culture where excellent care is a priority, patient safety is at the heart of concerns and every member of the team is valued.

5. Benefits for patients:
Strong clinical leadership results in better quality care, improved patient safety and a better overall patient experience.

6. Ongoing professional development:
Clinical leadership requires a commitment to personal learning and development. This could involve attending training courses, seminars or gaining further qualifications.

7. Challenges of clinical leadership:

Taking on a leadership role sometimes means facing resistance, managing conflicts and making difficult decisions. However, these challenges are also opportunities for growth and affirmation.

8. Mentorship and leadership:

Many nurse leaders stress the importance of having had a mentor to guide them on their journey. Conversely, as leaders, they have a responsibility to mentor the next generation.

Clinical leadership is an essential element in today's dynamic healthcare environment. For nephrology nurses, embracing this role can have a profound and lasting impact, not only on their careers, but more importantly on the quality of care delivered to patients. It is an invitation to be both a skilled clinician and a visionary, constantly seeking to improve the healthcare landscape.

Conflict management and promoting a positive working environment.

At the heart of the dynamics of hospitals and healthcare establishments, nephrology nurses are frequently confronted with stressful and sometimes conflictual situations. Managing these situations while fostering a calm and productive working environment is an art in itself, and an essential skill for the well-being of both professionals and patients.

1. Recognising conflict:

Before managing a conflict, it is crucial to recognise it. The signs can be subtle, such as a change in communication between colleagues or a palpable tension in the air, or more obvious, such as verbal disagreements.

2. Understanding the origins of conflict:
Conflicts can arise from many sources: differences of opinion, work-related stress, relationship issues or misunderstandings. Understanding them enables you to adopt an appropriate approach to resolving them.

3. Effective communication techniques:
Active listening, reformulation and open questioning are valuable tools for defusing a tense situation and understanding the other person's point of view.

4. Mediation as a solution:
In some cases, using a neutral third party to facilitate communication can help to find common ground and resolve the conflict.

5. Prevent rather than cure:
Setting up communication protocols, regular team meetings and training in conflict management can help prevent conflicts from arising in the first place.

6. Valuing diversity:
Teams are often made up of people from different backgrounds. Appreciating this diversity and understanding cultural or educational differences can contribute to a more harmonious environment.

7. Promoting well-being at work:
Relaxation areas, stress management training and recognition for a job well done all contribute to a positive working environment.

8. Constructive feedback:
Knowing how to give as well as receive constructive criticism is essential for professional growth and maintaining a healthy team dynamic.

9. The role of leaders:

Nurse leaders have a key role to play in creating a culture of respect, mutual support and open communication.

10. Continuous learning:

Seeing every conflict as an opportunity to learn allows us to grow professionally and strengthen the bonds within the team.

Conflict management and the promotion of a positive working environment are not just "soft" or secondary skills. They are fundamental to the smooth running of a nephrology unit, to the quality of care provided to patients, and to the mental and emotional well-being of professionals. In such a demanding field, creating and maintaining a calm working climate is a daily challenge, but also a reward in itself.

Chapter 14:
COMMUNITY RENAL HEALTH PROMOTION

Awareness programmes and prevention.

Nephrology, while central to the treatment of kidney disease, also plays a crucial role in preventing it. Awareness and prevention can significantly reduce the number of patients requiring heavy treatment, such as dialysis, and greatly improve the quality of life of many individuals. For nephrology nurses, these programmes are of vital importance, enabling them to act upstream and play an educational and preventive role.

1. Understanding the importance of prevention:
It is essential to understand why prevention is crucial. Detecting and treating kidney disease at an early stage can prevent later complications, save valuable medical resources and improve patients' quality of life.

2. Identify at-risk groups:
Certain groups, depending on their genetics, lifestyle or medical history, may be at greater risk of developing kidney disease. Targeting these groups can optimise prevention efforts.

3. Education and awareness:
Inform the public about the risk factors for kidney disease, its symptoms and the preventative measures they can take.

4. Workshops and seminars:
Organise educational events, where participants can learn, ask questions and benefit from preliminary screening.

5. Collaboration with other specialities:
Work jointly with specialists in diabetology, cardiology, and other fields, given that certain conditions, such as diabetes and hypertension, are risk factors for kidney disease.

6. Community-based interventions:
Establish prevention programmes targeting specific communities, taking into account their needs, culture and resources.

7. Setting up campaigns:
Use the media, social networks and other platforms to disseminate key prevention messages.

8. Training healthcare professionals:
Ensure that all healthcare professionals, not just those in nephrology, are well informed about best practice in preventing kidney disease.

9. Patient monitoring:
Establish a follow-up system for patients with risk factors, in order to detect any abnormality at an early stage.

10. Programme evaluation:
Regularly measure the effectiveness of awareness and prevention programmes in order to adjust them accordingly.

Nephrology nurses are not only key players in the treatment of kidney disease, but also in its prevention. Through awareness and prevention programmes, they can have a real and lasting impact on the kidney health of individuals and communities, while reducing the overall burden of kidney disease on the healthcare system.

The role of the nephrology nurse in community education.

Beyond the hospital setting, the nephrology nurse extends into the community sphere, playing the role of educator, guide and adviser. The importance of raising community awareness of kidney disease, its prevention and associated care is crucial to better public health management.

1. Public health educator:
Nephrology nurses have a wealth of information on the risk factors, prevention and treatment of kidney disease. As educators, they can organise seminars, workshops and presentations to inform the public about how to prevent kidney disease.

2. Community screening:
They can carry out screening campaigns in the community to identify people at risk or those starting kidney disease at an early stage, thus ensuring rapid and effective management.

3. Lifestyle advice:
The influence of lifestyle habits on kidney health is considerable. The nurse is able to guide the community on good eating habits, the importance of physical activity and the management of chronic diseases such as diabetes and hypertension.

4. Liaison with other health professionals:
The nephrology nurse may work in conjunction with other healthcare professionals, such as nutritionists or social workers, to provide comprehensive support to the community.

5. Promoting kidney health:

Awareness campaigns can be initiated or supported by nurses, highlighting the importance of the kidneys to general health and the measures to be adopted to ensure they function properly.

6. Psychosocial support:

Receiving a diagnosis of kidney disease can be overwhelming. Nurses can play a vital role in providing emotional support, answering questions and reassuring patients and their families.

7. Training and mentoring:

By training other nurses or healthcare professionals in nephrology, they ensure better dissemination of information and wider support for the community.

8. Cultural adaptation:

Each community has its own cultural particularities. Nurses must know how to adapt their messages and educational methods so that they are relevant and resonate with different audiences.

9. Family support:

By educating not only patients but also their families, nurses ensure a better understanding and management of the disease at home.

10. Post-hospital follow-up:

Discharge from hospital does not mean the end of the nurse's role. By providing follow-up in the community, they ensure that patients continue to receive the care and support they need.

The nephrology nurse is not just a hospital carer; he or she is a pillar of public health. Through community education, they play a crucial role in preventing kidney disease and supporting patients suffering from it. This extension of the nurse's traditional role highlights the versatility and importance of this profession in the global medical landscape.

Working with organisations non-governmental and patient associations.

Collaboration between nephrology nurses and non-governmental organisations (NGOs) and patient associations is a beneficial synergy for all concerned, especially the patients themselves. These interactions not only improve the quality of care and raise awareness, but also strengthen prevention and education programmes.

1. Awareness-raising and education:
NGOs and associations often have extensive networks and resources to run awareness campaigns. By working with them, nurses can reach a wider audience with accurate and relevant information about kidney health and care.

2. Patient support:
Patient associations often offer psychosocial support to people with kidney disease and their families. Nurses, in collaboration with these associations, can direct their patients to these valuable resources for further help.

3. Ongoing training:
Some NGOs offer training programmes for healthcare professionals. Nurses can benefit from these courses to improve their skills and keep up to date with the latest advances in the field of nephrology.

4. Prevention programmes:
By collaborating with NGOs that target kidney disease, nurses can participate in or initiate prevention programmes, such as community screening or vaccination campaigns.

5. Resources and materials:
Associations and NGOs can often provide material resources, guides, brochures or even medical equipment that nurses can use in their daily practice or to educate their patients.

6. Research and clinical studies:
Some NGOs are involved in research into kidney disease. By collaborating with them, nurses can take part in clinical studies, contribute to the development of new treatment methods or share their clinical observations.

7. Advocacy and lobbying:
With the support of powerful associations, nurses can engage in advocacy activities to improve health policies, obtain funding for research or advocate for higher standards of care in the field of nephrology.

8. Cultural and international exchanges:
Many NGOs operate internationally. Nurses can take advantage of these networks to exchange knowledge, practices and experiences with colleagues in other countries.

9. Networking:
Working with NGOs and associations offers nurses an excellent opportunity to network, build professional relationships and share ideas and resources.

10. Career development:
Nurses who actively collaborate with NGOs and

associations may also have the opportunity to progress in their careers, taking on leadership or management roles within these organisations.

The partnership between nephrology nurses, NGOs and patient associations is a win-win relationship. Each party contributes its skills and resources, leading to better patient care, increased awareness and an overall strengthening of nephrology care. These collaborations enrich the medical landscape and improve the lives of patients with kidney disease.

Chapter 15:
LEGAL QUESTIONS AND NEPHROLOGY

Legislation surrounding the practice of the nephrology nurse.

Nephrology, like all areas of medicine, is governed by precise legislation that sets out not only patients' rights but also the responsibilities and skills of healthcare professionals, including nurses. This legal framework guarantees not only the quality of care provided to patients, but also the safety of those providing it. It is therefore essential that all nephrology nurses have a thorough knowledge of these laws.

1. Qualifications and training:
The first legal concern is qualifications. To practise as a nephrology nurse, it is generally necessary to have undergone specific training after the nursing diploma and to be registered with a regulatory body.

2. Scope of practice:
The law clearly defines the scope of action of nephrology nurses: what acts they may perform, under what supervision, and under what conditions. This includes procedures such as accessing vascular lines, administering specific drugs, or monitoring during dialysis.

3. Liability:
Nurses, like all healthcare professionals, are legally responsible for their actions and omissions. They must practise with competence, diligence and integrity. Legislation also determines the extent to which they may be held liable in the event of professional misconduct.

4. Informed consent:
Before any intervention, the patient must give his or her consent. The nurse is often responsible for ensuring that the patient has fully understood the procedure, its benefits and risks, and the alternatives available.

5. Confidentiality:
The law imposes strict rules concerning the confidentiality of patients' medical information. Nurses must be vigilant to ensure the protection of this data, whether it is in paper, electronic or oral form.

6. Patients' rights:
Patients have fundamental rights that must always be respected, such as the right to dignity, respect for their person, the right to information, and the right to refuse treatment.

7. Working with other professionals:
The legislation also specifies how nurses must collaborate with other professionals, whether doctors, other nurses, dialysis technicians or social workers.

8. Clinical research:
If a nurse is involved in clinical research, he/she must be aware of the laws specific to human research, including consent, confidentiality and patient safety.

9. Continuity of care:
Legislation may also address the need for nurses to ensure continuity of care, even in the event of a patient transfer or change of team.

Legislation governing the practice of nephrology nursing is an essential component in guaranteeing safe, high-quality care. It is therefore vital for all nurses to keep abreast of legislative updates and developments, so that they can always practise in compliance with patients' rights and professional standards.

Patients' rights
and healthcare professionals.

In the medical world, the delicate balance between optimal patient care and respect for healthcare professionals is at the heart of daily concerns. Every individual, whether patient or healthcare professional, has fundamental rights that must be respected and protected.

As far as patients are concerned, the right to information is paramount. Every patient has the right to be informed about his or her state of health, the proposed interventions, and their potential benefits and risks. This enables them to make informed decisions about their treatment. This transparency, which is essential to respectful treatment, also implies the right to refuse treatment, to ask for it to be modified or to seek a second opinion.

However, information does not stop at the medical dimension alone. Patients also have the right to be informed of their rights, particularly with regard to the confidentiality of their medical data. All patients have access to their medical records and can request corrections if errors are identified.

Furthermore, the right to dignity and respect is fundamental. Whatever their state of health, social situation or origin, every patient deserves to be treated with dignity, without discrimination. This also includes the right to privacy and confidentiality, ensuring that intimate or sensitive details of their life and health are not disclosed without their consent.

As far as healthcare professionals are concerned, their rights often revolve around practising their profession in safe and dignified conditions. They have the right to ongoing training, enabling them to update their skills and provide quality care. They also have the right to work in a safe environment, where the risks of aggression or endangerment are minimised.

The right of expression is just as essential for professionals. They must be able to discuss, debate and express themselves on medical or ethical issues without fear of reprisal. This right goes hand in hand with their responsibility to report any act or situation that endangers the patient.

Collaboration is another aspect of the rights of professionals. Working in a team implies the right to collaborate constructively, to exchange relevant information about patients while respecting confidentiality, and to be able to count on the support of colleagues.

Respect for the rights of patients and healthcare professionals is a cornerstone of quality medicine. It is a delicate dance, in which each party takes care of the other, all in a common quest: the well-being and health of everyone.

Managing complaints and disputes.

The management of complaints and disputes is an inescapable aspect of medical practice. Any medical structure, whatever its degree of excellence, will be confronted, at one time or another, with complaints from patients or their relatives. These situations, far from being moments of failure, should be seen as opportunities for growth, learning and improving the quality of care.

1. Identify the source of the dissatisfaction.

The first step in dealing with a complaint is to understand its nature. Is it a communication problem, a disagreement about the treatment plan, a negative perception of the care received, or a genuine medical error? This understanding is crucial because it will guide the resolution process.

2. Active listening and empathy.

Listening is a powerful tool. Patients and their families often need to express themselves, to be heard and to have their emotions recognised. Empathy, the ability to put yourself in the other person's shoes and feel their emotions, is essential to defusing tension.

3. Provide clear answers.

Once the complaint has been clearly identified, it is essential to respond to it in a transparent manner. If a mistake has been made, it is essential to admit it, apologise for it and explain the measures taken to prevent it happening again.

4. Setting up mediation.

Some disputes may require the intervention of a mediator, a neutral person who will facilitate communication between the various parties and help them find common ground.

5. Accurate documentation.

Every complaint and dispute must be meticulously documented. This documentation must include the nature of the complaint, the people involved, the measures taken to resolve it and its outcome.

6. Systematic analysis.

Complaints must be analysed systematically, not only to resolve the current dispute, but also to identify any recurring patterns or problems. This analysis is a valuable source of information for the continuous improvement of care.

7. Training and prevention.
The best way to manage disputes is to prevent them. Ongoing training for professionals, the introduction of clear protocols and the promotion of transparent communication between patients and carers are all tools for reducing the risk of conflict.

8. Support for professionals.
Dealing with a complaint can be emotionally distressing for carers. It is therefore essential that they receive support, whether formal or informal, to deal with this ordeal.

Managing complaints and disputes is a complex process that requires careful listening, clear communication and a commitment to continuous improvement. In this delicate dance, patients and professionals move forward together, with the shared hope of an ever more efficient and respectful healthcare system.

Chapter 16:
CAREER DEVELOPMENT
AND CONTINUING EDUCATION

Specialisations in nephrology.

Nephrology, as a medical speciality focused on the kidneys and renal pathologies, offers a multitude of sub-disciplines for those wishing to further refine their expertise. These specialisations allow you to deepen your knowledge and skills in specific areas, ensuring optimal care for patients with special needs.

1. Renal transplantation.
This is a major sub-specialty that deals with the replacement of failing kidneys with a healthy kidney, usually from a donor. Professionals in this field coordinate the transplant process, from donor selection to post-operative care of the recipient.

2. Paediatric dialysis.
Paediatric nephrology is a specialisation focusing on the renal care of children from birth to adolescence. It deals with the unique renal pathologies of this population and how they interact with development and growth.

3. Interventional nephrology.
This speciality covers procedures used to identify and treat kidney disease without open surgery, such as catheterisation or renal biopsy.

4. Nephropathology.
This focuses on the microscopic study of kidney diseases

in order to establish a precise diagnosis and guide treatment.

5. Inherited kidney diseases.
This involves understanding and treating kidney diseases that are genetically transmitted, such as polycystic kidney disease.

6. Hypertension.
Although the management of hypertension is multidisciplinary, nephrologists are often involved because of the close relationship between blood pressure and renal function.

7. Critical nephrology.
This sub-discipline treats patients with acute renal failure or severe complications of chronic kidney disease requiring intensive care unit management.

8. Glomerulopathies.
This focuses on diseases that affect the glomeruli, the functional units of the kidneys responsible for filtration.

9. Renal lithiasis.
This specialisation covers the formation, detection and management of kidney stones.

Each of these specialisations, while remaining under the umbrella of nephrology, requires specific training and experience. They offer professionals the chance to deepen their knowledge, broaden their skills and make a significant contribution to medical science and patient welfare.

Nephrology research:
why and how to get involved?

Like other medical specialities, nephrology is constantly evolving, driven by scientific and clinical advances. Nephrology research is essential to improving our understanding of kidney disease, developing innovative treatments and improving patients' quality of life.

1. Why get involved in research?
   - **Improving patient care.** Research is often at the origin of new treatments, better diagnostic approaches and preventive interventions.
   - **Evolution of the profession.** Staying at the cutting edge of medical knowledge enables nephrology nurses to remain relevant in a changing medical environment.
   - **Contributing to medical knowledge.** Research is the tool by which medicine advances, and each study has the potential to make a significant contribution.
   - **Professional development.** Professionals involved in research can acquire new skills, gain recognition and develop their careers.

2. How can I get involved in research?
   - **Training.** If you're interested in research, it's essential to get some training, whether through courses, workshops or specialist diplomas. You need to master the ethical, methodological and statistical principles of research.
   - **Joining a research team.** Many hospitals and institutions have research departments or units. They can offer opportunities for collaboration, mentoring and direct involvement in research projects.
   - **Establishing collaborations.** Research is often a team effort. Collaborating with other professionals,

such as doctors, pharmacologists or biologists, can enrich a study.

- **Getting involved in clinical trials.** Nephrology nurses can play a central role in the implementation of clinical trials, from patient selection to data collection and analysis.
- **Taking part in conferences and symposia.** These events are excellent platforms for presenting work, getting feedback and networking with other research professionals.
- **Publishing and sharing.** Disseminating results is crucial in research. Publishing in scientific journals, presenting at conferences and even sharing on digital platforms are all ways of contributing to the global body of knowledge.

Getting involved in nephrology research offers the opportunity to make a significant contribution to the specialty and to patient health. It requires curiosity, determination and ongoing training, but the rewards, both professionally and personally, can be immense.

The importance of ongoing training.

In a world where science and technology are advancing at a breathtaking pace, the importance of continuing education for healthcare professionals, particularly those working in specialist fields such as nephrology, cannot be underestimated.

The dynamics of medical development
Nephrology, like so many other medical fields, is constantly evolving. New research is changing our understanding of kidney disease, innovative techniques are being developed for treatment, and new drugs are being introduced regularly. Without continually updating their knowledge,

nurses and doctors risk finding themselves out of date, potentially offering obsolete or less effective care.

Impact on the patient
A well-trained and well-informed professional is able to provide better quality care, inform patients adequately about treatment options and intervene rapidly in the event of complications. This translates into improved patient outcomes, fewer side effects and, in some cases, better survival.

Professional development
For nephrology nurses, continuing education is an opportunity for professional growth. It enables them not only to maintain and broaden their clinical skills, but also to explore new areas of specialisation or take on leadership or research roles.

Adapting to technology
With the introduction of new technologies in dialysis and other diagnostic tools, it is essential that professionals are trained in their optimal use. This goes beyond simply knowing about the machines; it means understanding how they fit into the patient's care pathway.

Building confidence
A professional who is actively pursuing his or her training is often perceived as being more committed to his or her profession. This strengthens the trust of patients and colleagues, encouraging better interprofessional collaboration.

Ethical and regulatory challenges
Nephrology, like other medical fields, is faced with ethical dilemmas, particularly when it comes to transplants, end-of-life decisions or new treatments. Ongoing training enables nurses to stay informed and prepared to navigate these delicate situations.

Continuing education in nephrology is much more than just a professional obligation. It is a reflection of nurses' commitment to providing optimal care, to developing professionally and to navigating the ever-changing medical landscape with confidence. By investing in their training, nurses are investing in their future, in the quality of the care they provide and, ultimately, in the lives and well-being of their patients.

CONCLUSION

The future of nephrology and the changing role of the nurse.

As the medical world moves forward, nephrology, like all specialties, is undergoing change, driven by research, technology and the changing needs of the population. This, in turn, is shaping and redefining the role of nephrology nurses, pushing them to be at the forefront of renal care.

Technological advances
The growing adoption of technologies ranging from telemedicine to advanced dialysis assistance devices offers unprecedented opportunities to improve the care of patients with kidney disease. Nurses, who are often the first users of these technologies at the patient's bedside, will become experts not only in their use, but also in training their colleagues and raising patient awareness.

The burden of chronic illness
With the increase in chronic diseases such as diabetes and hypertension, which are major causes of kidney failure, the need for nephrology care is growing. Nurses will play a central role in managing these diseases, preventing renal complications and educating patients about lifestyle changes.

Focus on prevention
As medicine moves towards a more preventative approach, nephrology nurses will be championing awareness and prevention of kidney disease. They will increasingly work upstream, educating communities and identifying people at risk long before symptoms appear.

Increased collaboration
The care of nephrology patients is complex and requires close collaboration between different specialists. In the future, nurses will play a pivotal role in coordinating care, working hand in hand with doctors, pharmacists, dieticians and other health professionals.

Progression to leadership positions
Recognising their unique expertise, nephrology nurses are expected to increasingly occupy leadership positions, whether in dialysis unit management, clinical research or health policy development.

Research and innovation
The role of the nurse will also extend into the field of research. They will be involved in clinical studies, testing new treatment methods, and will contribute to the science of nephrology through their observations and expertise.

The future of nephrology is bright and exciting. As the specialty continues to evolve, nephrology nurses are not just witnesses, but key players in this change. They will continue to be the backbone of patient care, while exploring new horizons, adopting cutting-edge technologies and playing an increasing role in shaping the future of renal care.

Glossary of commonly used medical terms.

Metabolic acidosis: A condition where the body produces excess acid or where the kidneys cannot remove enough acid from the body.

Anuria: Absence or extremely low production of urine.

Azotaemia: Increased concentration of nitrogen, particularly urea, in the blood.

Nitrogen balance: Measurement of the amount of nitrogen entering the body (mainly through dietary proteins) compared with the amount of nitrogen excreted in the urine.

Catheter: Flexible medical tube inserted into the body to administer or withdraw fluids.

Dialysate: Solution used in dialysis to eliminate waste products from patients' blood.

EPO (erythropoietin): Hormone produced by the kidneys that stimulates the production of red blood cells.

Arteriovenous fistula: Surgical connection between an artery and a vein, usually used for dialysis.

Glomeruli: Tiny filtering units in the kidneys where the blood is purified.

Haemodialysis: A type of dialysis in which the blood is cleaned outside the body using a machine.

Hyperkalaemia: High level of potassium in the blood.

Hypertension: High blood pressure.

Kidney failure: Inability of the kidneys to filter blood properly.

Nephron: Functional unit of the kidney, consisting of a glomerulus and tubules.

Nephropathy: kidney disease.

Osmolarity: Concentration of a solution, often used to describe the concentration of urine.

Polyuria: Production and excretion of a large quantity of urine.

Proteinuria: presence of abnormal amounts of protein in the urine.

Renin: Enzyme produced by the kidneys which plays a role in regulating blood pressure.

Kidney transplant: Surgical transplantation of a kidney from a donor to a recipient.

Uremia: High concentration of urea and other nitrogenous waste products in the blood, generally due to kidney failure.

Ureter: tube that carries urine from the kidney to the bladder.

Bladder: Term used to describe the bladder, an organ that stores urine.

This is an overview of the medical terms commonly used in nephrology. It is essential for all nephrology healthcare professionals to understand these terms in order to provide optimal patient care. This glossary can be expanded to include more specialised and technical terms, tailored to the needs of the specific readership.

Additional resources for learning and continuing training.

- Books and Manuals:
  - "Manuel de Néphrologie" by Dr. Jean-Paul Cristol and Dr. Philippe Brunet.
  - "The practice of haemodialysis" by Marc E. De Broe, Karl M. Koch, Norbert Lameire.
  - "Pathophysiology and diagnosis of kidney disease" by Robert W. Schrier.
- Professional journals:
  - Nephrology & Therapeutics.
  - Journal of the American Society of Nephrology (JASN).
  - Clinical Journal of the American Society of Nephrology (CJASN).
- Online training:
  - Coursera, Udemy and Khan Academy offer specific courses in nephrology.
  - Specialist websites such as Nephrology University or Renal Fellow Network.
- Professional organisations:
  - The French Society of Nephrology (SFN).
  - The American Society of Nephrology (ASN).
  - The European Renal Association (ERA).
- Conferences and workshops:
  - SFN annual congress.
  - Kidney Week organised by the ASN.
  - European meetings on nephrology organised by the ERA.
- Web resources and applications:
  - Medscape Nephrology: Latest news, studies and recommendations.
  - KDIGO (Kidney Disease: Improving Global Outcomes): Guidelines and recommendations

for the management of various kidney diseases.
  - NephroCalc: An application to help professionals assess kidney function and adjust medication.
- Podcasts:
  - "NephroTalk: Discussions on current topics in nephrology.
  - "NephJC": Reviews of relevant scientific articles in the field.
- Support groups and forums:
  - RenalWeb: Forum for dialysis professionals.
  - NephroLink: A platform for patients and professionals to exchange information and experiences.
- Resources for patients:
  - The Association for Information and Research on Genetic Renal Diseases (AIRG).
  - Kidney Foundation: Provides resources, information and support for patients with kidney disease.
- Specialised training programmes:
- Fellowship or specialisation programmes in nephrology offered by universities and hospitals.
- Medical databases and libraries:
- PubMed: Reference database for medical studies.
- Embase: Another essential resource for medical literature.
- Books and Manuals:
  - "Traité de Néphrologie" by Dr. Michel Paillard, Dr. Pierre Ronco, and Dr. Raymond Ardaillou.
  - "Nephrology for the nurse" by Maryse Aumont.
- Professional journals:
  - Nephrology & Therapeutics.
  - La Revue de Médecine Interne (founded by the Société Nationale Française de Médecine Interne).
- Online training:

- Université de la Francophonie: Specialised courses in nephrology.
- SIDES 3.0: Information system dedicated to teaching.
- Professional organisations:
  - La Société Francophone de Néphrologie Dialyse et Transplantation (SFNDT).
  - Association des Néphrologues Francophones de Belgique (ANFB).
- Conferences and workshops:
  - SFNDT annual conference.
  - Journées de Néphrologie (Nephrology Days): organised annually, these events cover a range of topics relating to the discipline.
- Web resources and applications:
  - NEPHROBLOG: Blog dedicated to nephrology, with numerous articles and information for professionals.
  - NéphroHUG: French-language portal dedicated to training in nephrology.
- Podcasts:
  - "NéphroScope": Discussions on current topics in nephrology for a French-speaking audience.
- Support groups and forums:
  - France Rein: Organisation working for the well-being of people affected by kidney disease in France.
- Resources for patients:
  - La Fondation du Rein: Organisation dedicated to information and prevention of kidney disease.
  - Info Rein: Information and exchange platform for kidney disease patients and their relatives.
- Specialised training programmes:
- Inter-university diplomas (DIU) in nephrology offered by various French-speaking universities.
- Medical databases and libraries:

- Banque de Données Santé Publique (BDSP) (Public Health Data Bank): Database containing a large number of documents in French relating to public health.
- BiblioSanté: Quebec platform offering reliable and relevant health resources.

Continuing education is essential for all healthcare professionals to ensure that the care they provide is based on the latest research and best practice. In nephrology, with technological and medical advances, keeping up to date is particularly crucial. These resources can help nurses and other professionals to continue their professional development.